TOXIC BY MIRANDA CAREY

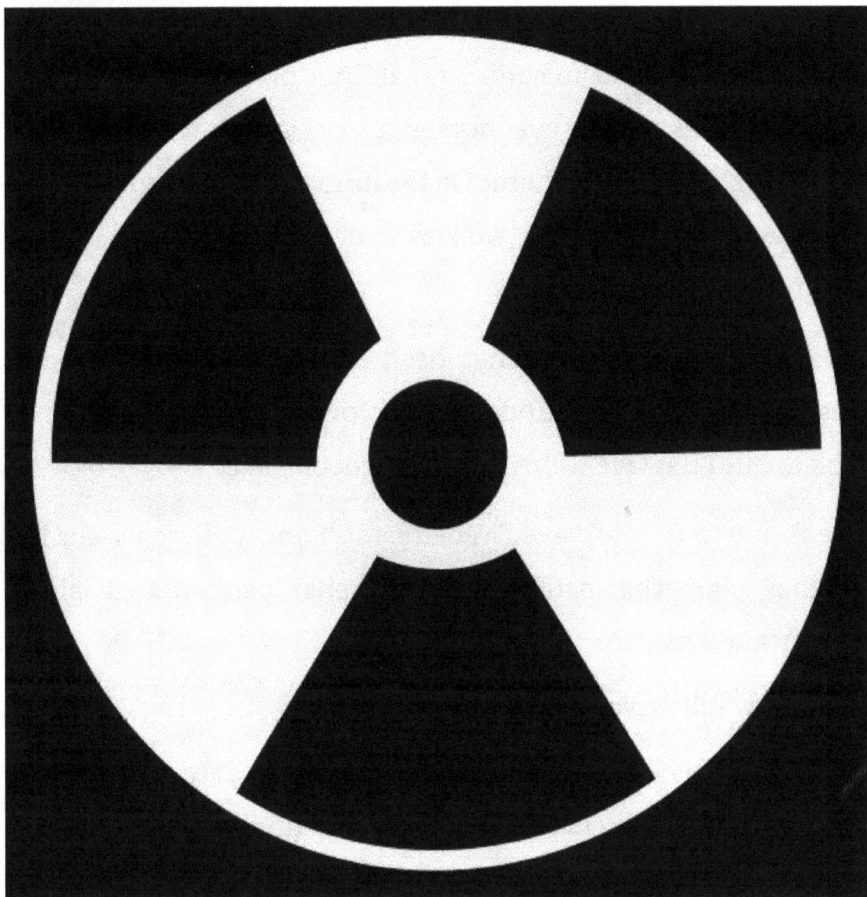

An Introduction to the Author

Miranda Carey is a qualified Nutritionist, Psychotherapist, Life Coach, and Magnet Therapist. A certified Holistic Health Practitioner with the AADP, American Association of Drugless Practitioners.

Ex professional 3-day event rider for Great Britain who lives in Spain where she had an equine rehabilitation centre and worked with charities for rescue horses and dogs. Now a full time practicing alternative therapist for humans and animals using bio magnetic therapy as well as a detoxification process for optimum health and fitness.

This 2nd edition of Toxic has been edited by my partner and Health Style Plus co-founder Steve Downs. Please take time to look at our Lifewave website and Facebook pages

Check out our LifeWave Website for Stem Cell rejuvenation patches, plus other patches for pain relief, performance, sleep, energy and skincare

https://www.lifewave.com/631435570

Health Style Plus for news, articles and up-to-date information on our other products and services including magnetic healing belts, magnetic jewelry, private health consultations and more

https://www.facebook.com/healthstyleplusfacebook

Discover the power of magnetic therapy, read about healing and treatments

https://www.facebook.com/MagneticTherapyHealth

Dedication

This book is dedicated to my parents, Peter and Pamela Carey, who have guided me through this muddle of a world and always backed me, even if they didn't agree with my choices, they have encouraged and supported my every move.

Foreword

Why did I write this book?

I wrote this book to make people aware that there are three things that cause disease and illness/poor health, barring accidents and surgeries. All are toxins that invade the body and leave catastrophic results. The different forms of toxins can be broken down into three basic categories.

1-POLLUTANTS

2-PARASITES

3-NEGATIVITY

What are they and where do they come from? I want to educate and inform you before you become ill. No-one wants to intentionally harm themselves, yet we do it daily without knowing.

This book will demonstrate to you how this is happening and help to reduce your load by showing you options and therapies.

There is a relationship between the mental outlook of a person and their physical state. Negativity and addiction can manifest themselves as illness in the body and mind.

Whilst there are many people already on the "health" bandwagon, the majority of the world are still believing advertisements on TV, and following the "what tastes nice" road, instead of looking at *why* they are ill, overweight, underweight, hurting, losing hair, teeth, becoming addicted, having to live on over the counter medication or prescribed drugs.

A lot of negativity derives from boredom... get a hobby, find a sport, play a game... find something to occupy your mind that you enjoy.

Why is there so much nastiness in the world nowadays? Why is there so much hate and aggression? The answer... toxins... confusing the brain and damaging the liver causing a huge combination of anger issues. People lose the ability to think rationally, with blocked up arteries/veins/blood vessels and tissues, stopping continuous blood flow to the brain.

Disease lives where there is a lack of oxygen. We will be looking at how to oxygenate the body in easy steps throughout the following chapters.

What inspired you to write Toxic?

I lived next to a children's hospital whilst I was growing up and couldn't believe the oncology ward being jammed full, these poor kids.

Given that most kids have a poor diet of processed and sugary foods, are exposed to chemicals daily in school, cleaning products in the home, car fumes, radiation, EMF and more we are only now understanding what all this really means to our families, it all starts when we are very young. Being aware of this inspired me to be as healthy as possible both on the inside and outside, in our home or when out and about.

My daughter inspires me to live healthily and to be able to do things with her. I wanted her to enjoy her mummy, living happy and well together, doing exciting things.

Having an aviary showed me how susceptible we all are to chemicals. The birds taught me not to use scented candles/chemical cleaners/Teflon pans or anything non-stick, anywhere in the house, they would keel over and die, so I considered, if it does that to them, what does it do to us??

The birds, my family and the dogs now only drink filtered, magnetized water. Removal of toxins became a way of life. My dogs now want carrots and apples as treats, and will not touch their old chemical loaded alternatives.

Horses and eventing played a huge part in my learning "another way". Riding for my country I was unable to use any form of drug to enhance performance or otherwise.

I set out to look for ways of getting the best out of my horses without putting them under any undue stress. The fitness routine for an event horse is crucial and rigorous. They need to be as fit as a racehorse, calm as a dressage horse and as careful as a show-jumper. They would show me what worked almost immediately, magnets being the wonder muscle relaxer, tendon cooler, and a Uric acid reducer after long exertion.

With eventing it isn't just the competition that's tough, it's all the preparation. Correct feed, good roughage, bedding, water, grooming, different forms of exercise for each different discipline, working on hard ground for tendons, soft ground because sometimes you had no choice, preparing in every way possible (breathing too) horse and rider fitness for the ultimate test of the three disciplines.

One of the great things with animals is you don't get the argument from their head, saying no I don't believe, you either see them get better or you don'. I saw results almost immediately with tendon issues, back problems, general well-being and sarcoids/sarcoma dropping off by using the zapper (see chapter 27)

I was a healthy event rider, very fit, thought I could do anything and survive it, having survived numerous falls; I felt I was SuperWoman.

This Super Woman then moved to the US, consumed an American diet, used well known creams, potions, soaps, scrubs and lotions, kept my household free from dirt and grime, washed my clothes in normal detergent and dishes the same, did everything, I thought, that was right for a healthy environment.

Unfortunately I also slept in a room with radios, PC, and TV which at the time I didn't know could cause disturbed sleep patterns, and other cognitive problems. Gradually over two years my health deteriorated, I put on weight, my joints hurt, I was continuously tired, sluggish, suffered from headaches, disturbed sleep....

I was being attacked from many different angles and the NEGATIVE people huff.....it's catching, it spreads like wildfire. It was all TOXIC.

Everyone I spoke to said ha! You're getting older now, this is what happens, go to the doctor and they will put you on some meds...???I don't think so... you accept that you are getting older so can't do things like you could before...NO WAY!

I decided enough was enough and set about extensive health research. I became aware of what to cut out like salt and sugar, I drank pure filtered, magnetized or distilled water, I ate as much raw, fresh food as possible, cut out meat and had very little dairy, I adapted my exercise regime, fasted where possible and made my own range of products for personal care and cleaning.

When in deep water paddle fast and build a boat!!!!

It was often said to me, "well I'm not giving that up because I like it"... .what a stupid thing to say, when you are ill because of it. I DO NOT MISS A THING, every now and then I get a craving, so I take extra potassium, zap or fast for a short time (24 hours to 3 days) after a 10 day fast, wow!, what a feeling. After the initial detox, what a high I had, a calm sense of well-being, my memory was fantastic, I was getting great sleep and energy...loads of it. I can smell well now too.

All my senses returned.

I wanted to show that even though there are lots of books on illness and diet fads and what you should do and not do, there was nothing that warned about the extras that we were consuming daily by means of environmental toxins, foods, drinks and personal care hazards. I loved my perfumes, creams and body baths, soaps, makeup, nail polish, extra conditioning shampoos and hair care, deodorant and scrubs...indulge??...not likely now I know the real deal. My own completely natural products keep my family toxin free from at least that part of life rather than pamper them in sheer luxury.

Another reason for writing was the latest trip to the supermarket, first of the month, welfare and food stamps are out. The fattest, most ill-looking, losing hair, no teeth collection of people are out in force to get their fixes....deli meats, baloney sausage in bulk, moon pies, bags and bags of candy, pop galore, they could hardly walk, could hardly get through the door....then needed the electronic shopping trolleys to sit on to get this grocery fix.

You can cheat a bit, but eventually you won't want to. The pure body is a great tool for being powerful, powerful in mind and body...able to achieve anything you set your mind to.

All Natural- What's that?

I didn't realise the significance of "all natural" and its importance in our lives until I started researching toxins and illness.

Natural, in this case literally means no nasties, no toxins, chemical-free, and non-harmful. Start with the soap you chose to put on your face and hands, choose all natural rather than one loaded with toxins and chemicals that will go through your skin, causing build up and harm to your body. Significantly reduce the intake of toxins by being natural, not hurting your skin and organs inside and out from constant commercial soap use, reduce effects like dry skin, dandruff, hair loss, acne ... .to name a few!!!

The damage takes a while, not at the beginning, when you first start using a product the chemicals seem to do you good , so you think hey this is ok, quick fix, after continued use the horrible stuff starts, organs affected, hair loss, skin that was becoming supple turns lined and haggard and loses elasticity etc., etc.

Natural products will cost slightly more than your mass produced chemically based ones, but they are cheaper in the long run, when you save on medical bills and healthcare, I think it's worth it.

If there is an ingredient name on a label you can't pronounce, DON'T USE IT... to eat, spray on the garden or put in the bath... READ LABELS!!!

This book only covers the basic causes of illness, for further information please seek a professional in the specific field.

Make time for health... convenience foods are a great excuse to say no time to cook, easier to grab a McDonalds...then look at the statistics of ill health worldwide, the worst hit areas? We can join the dots...exercise where possible...PRIORITISE!!!!

Get with a group if you can...strength in numbers.

I hope you enjoy this book, it will contribute to your wellbeing and that of others as you share the information provided.

Being aware is the key!

Quote "What does sugar do to the brain? It makes it mush ...."

No-one ever said a truer word!!!

Introduction

This book is certainly not designed to tell you to quit smoking or drinking right this minute, but we may make a mention of them in relation to other things. This book is intended as a guide to the toxins that we unwittingly put into our bodies daily, that make us ill, without knowing why.

Every illness and disease has a root cause from either a parasite or pollutant, or a combination, barring an accident.

All information in this book is thoroughly researched from various sources and is believed to be correct. It is not intended to be a cure or heal in any way, but to offer a different lifestyle and show the harm that chemicals and parasites do to the body, a look at how we can assist in their removal from our systems.

The importance of eating the right foods and eliminating toxins is linked to the brain and function of the whole body and its organs. Toxins can cause behaviour problems, autism, diseased and poisoned organs. Detox wherever possible to clean the system, mother nature and your body are remarkable working together to let you know in the form of flu/allergies/colds and illnesses...telling you that you need to stop and cleanse your body.

There is a zapper that you can use to eradicate and kill parasites at a vibrational level from your body, but the best thing, as with all this, is to clean what you put in, vegetables and fruit, I cleanse them with magnetic water, to get rid of pesticides and make them "live" food and a zappicator (www.zappertek.com) ... don't use cleaning materials with nasty chemicals, make sure your personal care is paraben free, sodium lauryl sulfate free and natural..

We, as a race of human beings nowadays, are toxic- in the air we breathe, tap water, car fumes, household cleaners, air conditioners, cigarette smoke, air fresheners in the chemicals we ingest through our food, pesticides, mineral oil, parabens, perfumes, shampoos, soaps, lotions, and detergents, to name but a few.

We touch things that have parasites and germs on, in shopping malls, on the carts, we have animals, we worm them, but do we worm ourselves..?

How do you avoid pesticides?...eat organic foods, if you can find foods that have not been in contact with any sprays, if so use the zappicator which will remove 90% of them. How do you avoid parasites? You simply can't. They are everywhere however you can minimize them by not bathing/swimming in lakes and rivers and by worming your animals regularly.

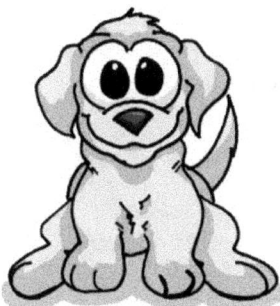

Solutions made with neem oil or apple cider vinegar are very effective for keeping fleas and ticks at bay from your pets, when sprayed on their coats, their beds, and all around your home. Diatomaceous earth too is very efficient for worming and as a flea control, be careful to only use food grade and watch for dust intake as you could damage their lungs and yours with inhalation.

Do not use antibacterial soap, as it contains more toxins than the damage you are trying to stop in the first place.

How does your body rid itself of toxins? Through the skin, urinary tract, liver, and bowels.

Sauna/steam room is good

Exercise is good

Sun is good (in moderation of course)

Signs of a Toxic body

The tongue is a real tell-tale sign of a toxic overload, if it is coated in white/yellow furry yuck, there is a chance you are highly toxic. Skin problems, spots, acne, not just on your face but can appear on your upper arms, back and chest. People with liver toxicity often have trouble sleeping, fatigue after eating, sugar, crash after a high, headaches to varying degrees, smelly urine, body odour, sinus problems, mucus and oral health. Smell sensitivity can mean you are overloaded with chemicals. Irrational moods combined with anger issues can be a major warning of liver toxicity.

The body has its own ways of filtering through the nasties but they will and do build up over time if the body is not allowed to get rid of them completely by fasting or other detox methods. It's not just our own body it's the earth, the magnetic field, air pollution, the weather patterns, our whole lives are being affected by TOXIC WASTE.

Most homes have a "kill corner" filled with all the worst chemicals possible, like roach killer, fly killer, household cleaners, detergents, fabric softeners, poisons and flea powders which contain formaldehyde, benzene and heavy metals that are all known carcinogens. You may have the "mother" that is the obsessive "cleaner" causing more toxicity and endangering the lives of the children and pets further. Flame - retardant in the sofa, solvents in carpets, cosmetics and glues.

We wonder why there are so many unhealthy, ill people (and pets) on this planet, these things that enter our bodies cause dizziness, cancers, brain diseases, reproductive harm and many awful unexplained illnesses that appear later on. A culling of the population.

Part 1 - Chapters 1-41
- Chapter 1 – What is happening to us NOWADAYS…
- Chapter 2 - Summary of an average daily chemical intake
- Chapter 3 - What toxins are found in commercial soap, deodorant, shampoo, beauty and cleaning products?
- Chapter 4 - Sugar, Addiction and Cravings
- Chapter 5 - Toxic Hunger
- Chapter 6 - Where hidden toxins live
- Chapter 7 - Low dose Cyanide exposure
- Chapter 8 - Bacteria
- Chapter 9 - Foods that feed parasites
- Chapter 10 - The Sun- signs of aging
- Chapter 11 - Pets
- Chapter 12 - Vaccinations
- Chapter 13 - Liver and anger issues
- Chapter 14 - Aspartame poisoning
- Chapter 15- Aluminium poisoning
- Chapter 16- Fertility
- Chapter 17- Mold
- Chapter 18- Sleep
- Chapter 19- Diabetes

CHAPTER 1

What is happening to us nowadays?

Years ago, we didn't have all these extra chemicals on our fruit and veggies, in our packets, a bag of flour, slab of butter and sugar might be what came from the store. Today we get all packet foods, everything preserved with x, y and z...

We get more colds than ever before, are filling up the hospitals and doctors surgeries with life threatening diseases, children have more learning difficulties, more people have diabetes and heart disease, cancer looms everywhere, more serious illnesses are popping up all the time. All these and more are due to toxic input.

You can blame who you like for becoming ill and feeling unwell, with the knowledge I show you in this book, you can make a change...it's up to you.

What goes into the body, what comes out of the body, exercise, rest, thoughts, everything you think and say...Like attracts like.

These areas have a direct relation to toxicity in the body, when you are toxic, your body is highly acidic, we need to be leaning towards alkaline in order to have a healthy body. Acidity creates illness and disease...every cancer patient has an acidic body.

Acidity derives from a bad diet, processed and packaged foods, drinking alcohol, smoking, sugar intake and unnecessary intake from air fresheners, car fumes, cleaning products in the home, even the water we bathe in.

We absorb toxins through our skin, like the ones used to grow fruit and vegetables, feed your chickens, feed the wildlife and water the trees.

You see what the knock on effect of toxins in your life can do, the air absorbs it causing catastrophic weather systems, earthquakes, volcanic eruptions and hurricanes/tornados, the earth's magnetic field is severely damaged again causing illness, as we lose our own magnetic fields due to pc's, cell phones, communication towers, radios, fossil fuels and more.

We can replace the magnetic field in each individual body by strong magnetic treatment. This is highly effective as no disease can live in a strong magnetic force. Drinking magnetic water is also very beneficial. It will help the detoxing process allowing the body's own systems to work harder at eliminating nasties.

There are magnetic insoles available and back belts along with necklaces, rings and eye masks to aid optimum health. Combining magnetic therapy with infrared which also aids circulation and healing.

Some of the most toxic working environments are mechanics, painters, cleaners and laboratory workers due to chemical exposure.

Highly likely too, that with heaters and fumes during the winter, people suffer from more disease, creating a breeding ground for toxins and bacteria.

Do you want to become another statistic?

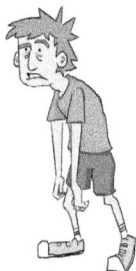

CHAPTER 2

An average DAILY INTAKE of chemicals, pollutants, toxins

1. Wash dishes
2. Do laundry

3. Shower/bath

4. Washing hands & Hand sanitizer (repeatedly in these times of covid-19)

5. Put on makeup/perfume/aftershave

6. Use hair spray/gel/mousse

7. Air con in car/house

8. Heating fumes

9. Air freshener

10. Toothpaste

11. Breathing in car fumes, walking in city smog

12. Preserved food

13. Fast food

14. Drinking soda

15. Smoking

16. Drinking

17. Go shopping, breathe in air freshener and cleaning products (bleach) from the shop

Whilst this is a list of what happens daily, you can reduce the amount by being careful and aware, the extras come from other places, listed in this book.

We all crave foods, thinking that we need it, telling ourselves by the clock, TIME TO EAT, FILL UP NOW, Just another way to toxic overload - organ wear-out, we all eat too much plus drink the toxic beverages as a way of life, those who still smoke and external chemicals we add in shampoos, soaps, creams etc.

It's no wonder most people are not living out their true lifespan, but cutting it short and suffering through medications. If they would only look at the whole picture, what has caused this? Can this be reversed? The answer....YES it can...

CHAPTER 3

What Is in commercial soap, Deodorant, Shampoo?

Beauty products & Cleaning Products

Methyl, Propyl, butyl and ethyl parabens- Used to preserve the shelf life of products, they are highly toxic, carcinogenic (cause cancer) and cause skin conditions.

Synthetic colours, as with food colours, these go by names like... F, D & C or D & C followed by a number. They are known to cause cancer, even toothpaste and toothbrushes contain these harmful ingredients. The coloured toothbrush contains the dyes which are absorbed through the mucus membranes in the mouth and into the bloodstream...

Petrolatum - Mineral Oil and Jelly that promotes sun damage and leads to dry skin and chapping as well as skin conditions. Found in petroleum jelly and baby oil amongst many others.

Sodium Lauryl Sulphates - Used in shampoo, body wash and soap to make lather. It also causes skin conditions, hair loss, eye irritations, dandruff and allergic reactions.

Imidazolidinyl urea and diazolidinyl urea (Germall II and Germall 115) - commonly used preservatives in many personal care products and cosmetics causing skin conditions. The latter releases formaldehyde when it is above 100 degrees F.

PVP/VA copolymer- A petrochemical used in hair spray, perm solutions and many cosmetics. The particles may stay in the lungs, causing respiratory problems.

Stearalkonium chloride- Used in hair-conditioners and skin creams, this is a toxic ingredient developed by the fabric industry originally as a fabric softener...yes that means fabric softeners are toxic too.

Fragrance/perfume- up to of 3000 chemicals, mostly derived from petrochemicals, this causes discolouration of the skin, headaches, asthma, joint pains, muscle pain, fatigue, swollen lymph nodes, raise blood pressure, dizziness, rashes, skin irritation and coughing to name a few!!! Only essential oils do not have this, any fragrance oils are lethal, make your own perfume with your favourite oil/combination of oils mixed with a nice carrier oil.

Dioxin- A known carcinogen, dioxin is used in toilet roll, kitchen roll/paper towels plus many feminine hygiene products such as tampons and pads. Dioxins absorb through the skin and are linked to immune disorders, endometriosis and cancer of the reproductive system.

Fluoride- Excessive amounts of fluoride are linked to cancer and brain problems, found in toothpaste and most tap water.

Coal tar- Found in most hair dyes, coal tar is linked to numerous types of cancer, including non-Hodgkin's lymphoma.

Lead- A heavy metal linked to brain disease and many other illnesses, lead is commonly found in lipsticks.

Cleaning Products

Benzene - linked to cancer (predominantly leukemia) and in the male reproductive system.

Chloroform - causes cancer and development toxicity

Dibutyl Phthalate - damages male and female reproductive systems

Air Fresheners - this covers bottled, canned, plug-ins and sanitizers. Avoid inhaling spray mist or vapour!!!

Acetone - This is a blood, heart, gastrointestinal, liver, kidney, skin, respiratory, brain and nervous system toxin.

Butane and isobutene - Lighter fuel!!! Serious brain and nervous system toxins...

Liquid petroleum gas and petroleum distillate- air fresheners/car fresheners...

Propane - this is a cardiovascular and blood toxin as well as a liver, kidney, respiratory, skin and nervous system toxin known to be highly dangerous.

Benzene - as above linked to leukemia.

Formaldehyde - as above plus linked to cancers of the upper airways.

Overwhelming, yes, to learn that so many of the foods, beauty products and household products we've come to rely on- are fully toxic.

We wonder why we are becoming old before our time..!!!

Go Natural!!!!

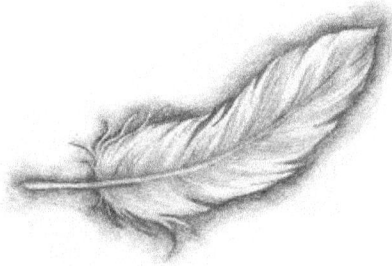

CHAPTER 4

Sugar, addiction and cravings...

Dangers of sugar are now linked to Alzheimer's, diabetes, autism, liver damage, arterial damage, heart disease, the blocking up of the whole system causing brain fog, accelerated aging, memory loss, Candida, yeast overgrowth and fungi build up. It feeds and fuels diseases of all types, parasites and fungi feed off it and thrive.

Sugar can cause dementia and liver damage, anger issues, pancreatic problems, and aging skin.

When the arterial veins are blocked the brain is deprived of the correct amount of blood, creating confusion, stroke, creating addiction with the hypothalamus's inability to send correct messages from the brain to the bodily function. The cortex gains fungi, more confused thoughts, cravings and irritability also blocking the vena cava and aorta, the main vein and artery into the heart.

Sugar is disguised as dextrose, sucrose, lactose, high fructose, starch and carbohydrates. They are found in pasta, soda pop, milk, bread, processed foods, meats, packet foods, tinned foods, cakes, pastries, and cereals.

These all create dopamine in the brain and reward the body with a good feeling, a "high" which doesn't last for long developing a "crash" as the effect wears off, exactly the same as for heroin, cocaine, nicotine, alcohol and other recreational drugs. Over the counter meds can cause a similar feeling, creating a major psychological problem on top of the addiction. Childhood candy can cause anorexia, bulimia, drug abuse, smoking, alcoholism, obesity and depression.

Be sensible and realize what sugar is doing to your children, they will not miss it if it's not given to them, and will be so much more healthy, it is only you that thinks that are suffering by not having sugar. At kid's parties where sensible foods are given, everyone plays together, no fighting, all happy and harmonious. Kids parties with high sugar content always ends in tears, fighting, jealousy, screaming and crying.

This addiction that starts in childhood by eating a lot of sweets, candy, chocolate, chocolate milk (dairy and sugar together, like ice cream is even worse) it's teaching a bad habit from an early age which may lead to smoking cigarettes and drinking soda... and it goes on from there, linked also to crime and jail, hoarding and...obsessive disorders.

The only good use for sugar is in a scrub!!!

Addicts like to feel in control of their situations and surroundings, so their sense of control as a bulimic is in secret, no-one knows what they are doing but they are in control of their body and it feels good. Simulated by the nicotine high, the chocolate rush for example, this control feeling is also brought about in relationships, drug abuse/use.

Addicts cannot stop themselves, they think they are not doing anything wrong, just using a situation to suit themselves and until they can see there is a need for help, or their bodies tell them, hey you are toxic, no one can help them, everyone seems against them, it's not their problem but everyone else's, they go on pretending it doesn't exist, so they can continue with their destructive lifestyle.

Toxic people...how they behave: Drug use and abuse, blaming others, greed, theft, crime, ego, materialism, controllers, and dictators.

See how one little sugar lump made a monster!!!

CHAPTER 5

Toxic Hunger

The hunger that happens when your digestive system stops working, making your other organs work instead to cleanse the body...your body has to stop the digestive system working in order to assist the other organs in the clean out, it cannot detox whilst processing food, so you feel hungry..

The hunger you experience is controlled by eating a little, which in turn sets the digestive system off again...stopping the detox... so you feel hungry only when you are in a state of detox/fasting. When you eat, the detox stops and concentrates on the digestive systems again, making the other organs now work harder to get rid of chemicals from the body. Why when fasting you can experience undesirable symptoms as other organs clear out their bad stuff.

This is a temporary state and can be quite beneficial to the body to complete the clean out.

CHAPTER 6

Where hidden toxins live

In children's toys, the rubber/plastic is made with phthalates (plasticizers)...highly toxic, where do kids put most toys? In their mouths...immediate ingestion of chemicals through osmosis, plus bits chewed off.

Plastic food and drink containers that contain BPA and PET, all highly toxic chemicals that are in the plastics, which subsequently leak into the beverage or food, worse when heated up, in a hot car, or microwave.

In feminine care...Tampons, sanitary towels and underwear.

Synthetic fibers, chemically-soaked cotton, petrochemical and plastic additives, hazardous odour neutralizers and fragrances, and rayon that is chlorine-bleached (a process shown to release cancer-causing dioxin and other by-products), can also cause fertility problems, the same chemicals are used to make baby's diapers.

Talcum powder is known to contain horrendous chemicals that cause ovarian cancer, damaging the reproductive system and drying out the skin, baby powder too.

Baby oil contains mineral oil which comes from petroleum.

Toilet-rolls and paper towels, the same as for feminine care.

Clothing, yes, in your own clothes from the dyes and formaldehyde.

Toothbrushes, all the colours that look pretty are in fact dyes that cause toxic bodies, look for bamboo and natural bristles.

Microwave ovens, emitting electro-magnetic field radiation, are radioactive.

Food dyes, from kids' parties, most packet foods.

Monosodium Glutamate is found in most packet foods, Chinese food and spices to name but a few.

Radon - A natural radioactive gas that can seep into homes through cracks in the walls, it enters the body through inhalation.

Carbon Monoxide- from burners, propane, butane and oil.

Vinyl chloride - the "new car" smell, plastic of a new car gives off this chemical.

CHAPTER 7

Environmental Cyanide Exposure/intoxication

This is all around and uncontrolled, entering food, water supplies, the air.

Low-dose exposure results in allergies, cold and mucus symptoms, bronchitis, asthma, and irritated eyes.

Inhalational exposure results in shortness of breath and breathing difficulties, cough, and chest discomfort. People are completely unaware that they may have this in their bloodstream and organs...

Two of the antidotes are Sodium Thiosulfate Pentahydrate which can be taken with great success under supervision for correct dosage and Alpha-Ketoglutaric Acid, a natural organic acid.

'The Poisoned Planet' by Timothy Oesch is available on kindle from Amazon. This book is extremely informative about the detoxification from highly toxic substances.

CHAPTER 8

Bacteria

Bacteria is everywhere, transferring from place to place causing streptococci and Staphylococcus h pylori...the worst place for it to occur is in the kitchen on towels and sponges, where bacteria breeds in the warm humidity...wash and dry all sponges frequently, clean cutting boards, kitchen surfaces, sink drains, doorknobs , toothbrushes by sterilizing equipment, vinegar, bicarbonate of soda, borax. H2O2.

Sponges and rags pass the dust and eggs of tapeworms and roundworms, bug bits and other nasties which spread from surface-to-surface, onto mugs and glasses, plates, knives and forks directly into the body.

It is a good idea to have an electric sterilizer that heats everything to high temperatures, no bug or worm egg can survive, failing that, spray H2O2 or Dettol on surfaces and use a clean sponge to wipe them down.

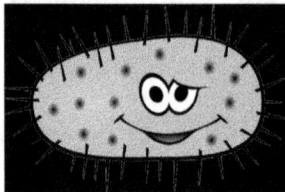

CHAPTER 9

Foods that feed parasites

The number one food that parasites feed on is sugar. This includes all forms of processed sugar and artificial sweeteners. Sodas too, along with energy drinks, commercially packaged fruit drinks, candy, processed chocolate and other sweets.

Baked goods also contain sugar. These include cakes, pies, cookies and even breads. Pastas, cereals and others that easily convert to sugar also feed the parasites. Basically, anything that is made with white flour will provide an environment for the parasites to thrive in.

Unhealthy fats are another food that parasites love to feed on. These fats are vegetable oils and animal fats. Processed foods such as chips, prepared frozen meats and French fries, are often loaded with high amounts of unhealthy fats.

All meats, dairy and dairy products as well as eggs contain unhealthy fats that feed parasites, and thus should be eliminated from the diet.

Some fruits also contain high amounts of sugar, and thus they tend to feed the parasites as well. Other fruits however, such as papaya, pineapple and tomatoes have been shown to help eliminate parasites.

By eliminating these foods from your diet you are well on the way to getting rid of the parasites from your body, without the feeding routine the parasites will die off.

CHAPTER 10

The sun and aging process

Sun is good, it is your friend, providing you with vitamin d...it brings out toxins...known as WRINKLES....don't be dismayed at these, at least they are not in your body...spots and acne, rashes are all tell-tale signs that your body is overloaded with toxins.

How to reverse these signs of aging?

Drink copious amounts of water, use magnets daily like those in insoles, juice, eye masks, use all natural foods and personal care, drink magnetic water, use it on your plants too, they thrive on it!!! Animals too benefit enormously from magnetic water. Birds, dogs and cats will instinctively be drawn to it, they know that it will improve their overall health.

Eat a good balanced diet of mainly organic veggies and fruit, cut down on dairy and meat, these slow the system down, taking days instead of hours to digest, taking unnecessary pressure to the rest of the organs, making them all work harder. Unclog the arteries/veins/capillaries that lead to heart disease, strokes, fibromyalgia, arthritis, diabetes, autism, ADHD, poor eyesight, poor hearing etc., etc. Everything can be reversed, if you want to do it. Premature aging can and will be reversed if you cut out/reduce sugars and salts, solid fats and preservatives, food dyes and other harmful toxins.

At this point of the book, I would recommend that you check out our LifeWave website to find out more about the Stem Cell stimulating patches that we use on ourselves and our animals https://www.lifewave.com/631435570

CHAPTER 11

Pets

By using common household cleaners, you could be slowly poisoning your dog without even knowing it. You could be putting your pet at risk of developing cancer, kidney or liver damage. Studies have proved the toxic effects of such ingredients as ammonia, bleach, chlorine, glycol ethers and formaldehyde on humans and pets.

Pets pick up residues from cleaning products, carpets, air fresheners and then groom themselves, spreading these toxic materials on their skin, coat, mouths, nose and eyes. Toxic materials also come from garden sprays.

Avoid using any commercial shampoos for your pets and flea collars/powder, chemical bug repellents as these affect the liver and brain of your pets shortening their lives considerably.

Flea & tick control...use Neem Oil in a natural shampoo, apple cider vinegar diluted spray helps all skin conditions.

Feed carefully, checking ingredients for preservatives, chemicals and dyes...birds, especially, are given sugar treats as "pellets" that are, so say, good for them, then linked to diabetic birds and obesity, fatty liver disease, better to make your own with all natural ingredients.

There are natural worming methods you can use for your pets.

Amazing results have been seen using our Lifewave Stem Cell activation patches to treat all kinds of illnesses and health issues for pets.

Find them here: https://www.lifewave.com/631435570

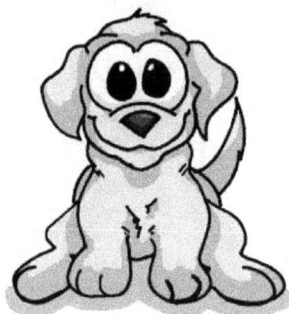

Worming recipe

For the first week, 1 teaspoon of parsley water on their food.

Second week, parsley water, same measurement and black walnut tincture 1 drop on food.

Third week, parsley water, black walnut tincture and a pinch of wormwood powder.

Fourth week, parsley water, black walnut tincture, wormwood and pinch of cloves on food.

Don't force your dog/cat to eat this as any bit they consume will be beneficial to killing off the parasites.

Diatomaceous earth is also a very good parasite control for animals and humans, only food grade is safe to use and is available from Amazon.

NEVER give the rawhide chews and treats as they are carcinogenic, filled with chemicals and can cause severe illness, plus risk choking them, the poor pet doesn't know any better and is totally in our hands to feed, water and treat as we wish....READ LABELS AND DO YOUR RESEARCH.

CHAPTER 12

Vaccinations

These are causing no end of health problems, by directly giving the disease to inoculate ... .warnings of high fever, malaise, brain problems, sight, headaches, a dose of the disease may not be so good, can be fatal if not kept under supervision for the first few days. Glyphosate has been found in children's vaccines, a known toxic pesticide, and Aluminium which comes with its own horror stories.

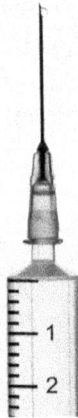

Image by rawpixel.com

CHAPTER 13

The liver and anger issues

Your liver is the largest organ that deals with detoxing your body, which means all the chemicals and parasites go through this dead or alive. The liver stores nasties for you if it can't clear it to be passed, causing major toxic overload Toxins get "stuck" in the liver, and depending on how full it is as to how angry the person becomes, this can be quite overwhelming and uncontrollable until dislodged.

When we get that awful feeling of not being able to understand why you feel so at odds with the world and just so cross... blaming anyone for everything, rest assured it's the liver bunged up.

These toxins/chemicals mainly come from smoking, taking drugs and eating a bad diet of junk/tinned/processed food.

This connection has been observed in prisoners, people who spend a good deal of their existence living the junkie's life, drugs and food...habits that form....dysfunctional expression of anger.

Milk thistle, which is related to the daisy family, has a long history of being used medicinally for healing. It's well known for helping any and all types of liver problems and is said to be good for detoxing from chemical overexposure.

There are many different liver detoxes that can be used, but by far the best is the fasting, firstly by juice fast, then gradually detoxing from other regular foods/chemicals , caffeine, fluoride, sugar, nicotine, alcohol, etc. , giving the body a rest to get these "stuck" toxins out..

CHAPTER 14

Aspartame poisoning

This is becoming the new lethal drug ... .found in diet drinks, sugar-free products, in packets, cereals, yogurts...misleading that it is healthy...extremely acid forming, it affects every part of the body in a different way, attacking the body as a whole.

The aspartame in diet drinks breaks down into the same properties as embalming fluid.

Aspartame causes nerve damage, headaches, dizziness, neuropathy, loss of feeling in limbs, pins and needles...muscle damage.., abdominal pain, bloating and gas, menstrual cramps, fluid retention and excessive thirst, high blood pressure, asthma like symptoms, ringing in the ears, loss of taste, painful swallowing,

it can also cause severe depression as it affects the brain psychologically, as well as causing memory loss and mood swings.

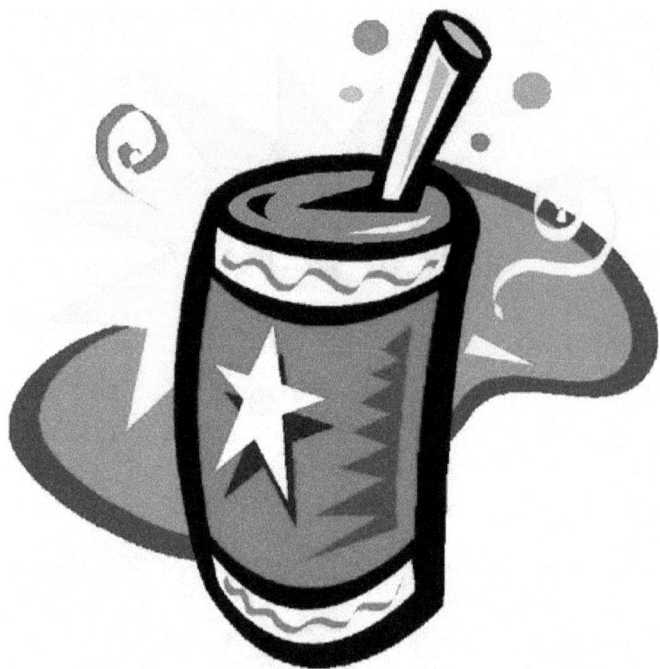

CHAPTER 15

Aluminium poisoning

You can find Aluminium in deodorant and douches, in food additives such as those in cake mixes, frozen dough, self-rising flour, processed cheese and cheeseburgers ... .having one of the highest contents of Aluminium. Cooking with Aluminium pots, using foil wrap and it is found in over-the-counter medications.

Aluminium causes aching muscles, speech problems, kidney, liver, digestive problems, anemia, and reduces bone density. It can cause problems with the nervous system, including disturbed sleep, emotional problems, memory loss and headaches.

CHAPTER 16

Fertility

Some diseases, like polycystic ovary syndrome and endometriosis may even stem from early toxin exposure.

Make sure you use cotton underwear and natural sanitary towels/douches/tampons.

Toilet roll, tampons and sanitary towels contain chlorine/dioxin which is a nasty chemical that causes a lot of problems with the female reproductive system. Talc is known to cause ovarian cancer and inhibit male organs. Use natural soaps and coconut oil/Epsom salts to bathe in.

A good detox is necessary if you think you have had a chronic toxic overload before becoming pregnant, to aid the pregnancy, the birth as well as the child and mother.

CHAPTER 17

Mould

Mold emits toxins that the body must detoxify. These substances, known as volatile organic compounds or VOCs, produce the musty odor of mold. Some of the gasses produced include hexane, benzene, acetone and methylene chloride.

Aflatoxins may be present in many different types of foods. This includes cereals, tree nuts, corn, peanuts/peanut butter, pistachios, Brazil nuts, chilies, black pepper, dried fruit and figs. Milk, cheese, and dairy products may be contaminated with aflatoxins.

Mold has been linked to the AIDS epidemic.

Corn is probably the commodity of greatest worldwide concern, because it is grown in climates that are likely to have perennial contamination with aflatoxins and corn is the staple food of many countries.

Black Mold causes chronic sinusitis, headaches, dry, itchy eyes and skin rashes.

CHAPTER 18

Sleep

Beauty sleep has a new meaning...as your brain and body detoxes during sleep. Lack of sleep impairs brain function leading to children's learning difficulties and many illnesses in general, as the body is unable to fully repair itself without the sleep needed.

Try to relax and unwind before going to bed, listen to soft music or read something soothing. Try to not watch nasty or action movies as they will impede the quality of sleep, much needed for the brain and bodily cleanse. Use magnets to sleep for sound, relaxed quality sleep.

Sleep apnea is caused by blockages and obstructions/toxins in the airways and veins from the heart to the head. This condition can be lethal when the heart stops and starts when blockages are more severe. Detox the body from the chemical and parasitic obstructions.

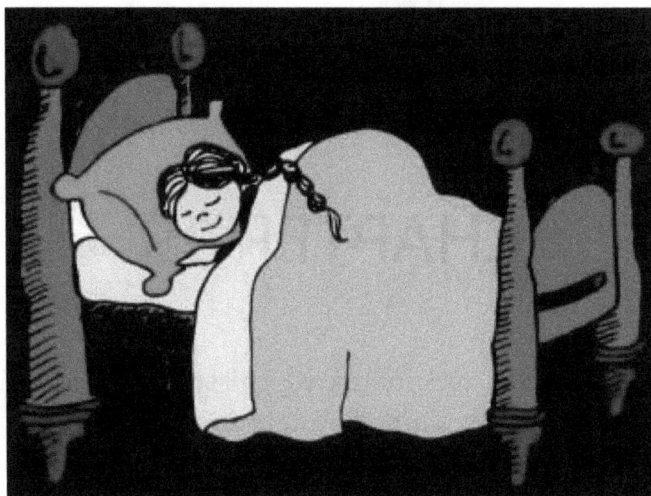

CHAPTER 19

Diabetes

Diabetes symptoms are increased thirst, frequent urination, extreme hunger, unexplained weight loss, fatigue, irritability, blurred vision, compromised immune system making sores slow to heal...to name but a few.

It has been found now that not only was the sugar causing problems, it was arsenic and dioxin levels too...

Arsenic is found in make-up, marine foods, drinking water, some drugs, wood preservatives and pesticides.

Dioxin is found in beef, milk, chicken, pork, fish and eggs, also diapers, sanitary care, toilet roll and paper towels.

Use Stevia as a sugar substitute, juice, fruit and vegetables to oxygenate the cells reducing the level of acidity in the bloodstream.

Use magnets where possible and drink magnetic water to flush the body and aid optimum blood flow to extremities, especially fingers and toes.

CHAPTER 20

Asthma

Asthma is on the rise with so many cleaning products and personal care products, air fresheners on the market, linked with hormone disruption and severe breathing difficulties.

Products that may cause bad reactions are cat litter, imagine what it does to your cat? Diapers, glass cleaners, floor cleaners, shampoo, conditioners, dish detergent, laundry detergent, toothpaste, deodorant, mascara, shower curtains , dryer sheets, sunscreens, perfumes and nail polish.

The fumes we are exposed to... walk into most shops and you are bombarded with air freshener and bleach "clean" smells, car fumes, air conditioners, kerosene heaters, the list is endless. These all trigger asthmatic symptoms, use of a humidifier can reduce symptoms. Drink good filtered water only, magnetic water is even better.

CHAPTER 21

Autism

Just a few years ago, autism affected 1 in 10,000 children. Nowadays it is becoming increasingly bad, affecting more like 1 in 50.

Fluoride alone can contribute to a large drop in the IQ of a child. Genital malfunction is also a symptom that can be brought on by over exposure to toxins. Fluoride was used in concentration camps during the war to get prisoners to cooperate, by dulling their senses...impairing their brain function.

Parents that smoke, homes that have heating fumes throughout the house, cleaning products, drug use, all of these contribute to an over exposed toxic home.

Glutamine, found in dairy products and meat, can contribute to fueling this illness, soy is high in glutamine...found in baby formula and can cause psychiatric disorders, kidney and liver disease.

CHAPTER 22

Allergies

The same as the other illnesses, overly toxic bodies can't cope with extra toxins so it shows up as an allergy.

Detoxify yourself, detoxify your home (cleaning products, personal care products, air fresheners) and lifestyle (your diet) and your allergies will go away.

Trial and error as to which works quicker and has the most effect (everybody is different and has to be treated as such) mono foods, eat one food for a while to see if that affects you, whilst clearing all other toxins from the home, the car, office.

Use a humidifier in the home/office. Put moisture into the air you breathe with good filtered water.

CHAPTER 23

Hair loss

Hair loss can be caused by a number of factors, but usually a combination of chemicals – Your shampoo and conditioner, plus parasites are enough to create havoc within the hair follicle and scalp.

Using Bentonite clay in your shampoo can help restore and detox, neem oil, coconut oil for parasite removal and diatomaceous earth will help with detoxing from heavy metals.

Hormones can also cause problems normally from being toxic, nutritional factors also play a big part.

Candida and sugar cause problems, parasites feeding from the sugar in the body, thriving on it and growing, blocking up arteries, follicles, capillaries, veins.

Vitamin and mineral deficiencies in B vitamins, magnesium, zinc, iron can have a drastic effect on hair loss too.

CHAPTER 24

Garden Care

As you want your body to heal and be well from toxic overload, your garden plays a HUGE part in this.

Glyphosate – exposure to and what you spray on your weeds and keep mosquitoes and bugs away with, also enter your body, your child's and pets, plus birds and bees in your garden, look for all natural pesticides...neem oil diluted with water, citronella with water, have a bug zapper outside that doesn't emit deet and other chemicals.

The insect repelling coils you can burn are lethal, with 4000 different chemicals entering the air as they smolder away, scented candles too...even unscented candles give off chemical waste. Use tea lights and essential oils for a fresher safer home, inside and out.

Toilet cleaner/bleach gets absorbed into the garden, into rivers and the earth which in turn cause the overheating of the ozone layer, creating bad weather, plus the damage it's doing to the wildlife, plants that we eat, in the vegetable garden, fruit trees, the meat and fish caught for consumption.

CHAPTER 25

Anxiety

A diet of fried foods, alcohol, coffee and dairy products can all cause the liver to overwork and struggle with feelings of anger/anxiety. Dairy products raise the adrenaline levels which contribute to a more anxious feeling. Fried foods being hard to digest put extra pressure on the other cleansing organs causing temporary feelings as they are passed through. Pesticides increase the rate of depression, make sure you wash your veggies well in magnetic filtered water, if available, or use an ozonator.

Don't use chemical bug repellents, flea treatments or flea shampoos on your pets or you will both be poisoned too. They affect the brain and livers of both you and your pets, shortening their life span… and yours!

See also gluten intolerance.

CHAPTER 26

Candida

Poor diet fuels this horrible disease, and wreaks havoc within the body...Sugar, dairy products (milk especially- lactose) and refined white flour(bread , cakes, candies) feeds the fungi and yeast overgrowth which escalates within the body causing tiredness, itchy skin, stomach pain and digestive problems, brain fog, anxiety, anger, headaches, cravings, acne, irritability and mood swings.

Antibiotics, birth control pills, steroids, antacids...these all contribute to this nasty disease.

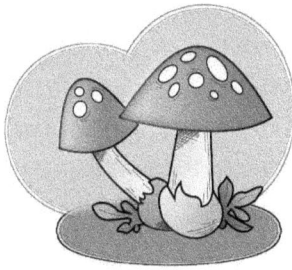

CHAPTER 27

Parasites

Where do they come from?

Fruits and vegetables that haven't been washed properly ,undercooked, raw fish, meat and poultry, polluted soil and water, poor hygiene, increased international travel to third world countries...rats and mice, airborne, ticks...your supermarket buggy/trolley...public toilets....dust that travels through the air bringing tapeworm, roundworm eggs galore into your home, airways, wiped down on surfaces, entering your body.

What do they cause?

Joint and muscle pain, gas and bloating, diarrhea, anemia, allergies, growths such as cysts and tumors, non-malignant, skin complaints, nervousness, respiratory problems, sleep problems and tooth grinding, constipation where the parasites block the intestines, fatigue, obesity, immune system problems, excessive hunger, bad breath, epilepsy and migraines..

These parasites also have their own toxins, their urine and feces, which in turn cause us more toxicity. They also eat through stomach linings and tissues, muscles in the body causing fluids to leak into the blood, digestive, uriary, lymphatic, blood fluids, peritoneal fluids...all causing much like a 24 hour flu symptom...but worse, can cause recurring allergies and bodily swelling (edemas)

Feasting on our nutrients, starving the body of what it needs to survive, creating disease.

By continual detoxing, fasting, you can eliminate these worms and parasites ...by also using a zapper, designed by Hulda Clark...and or ozonator/zappicator which cleans the fruit and veg before you eat it...www.hulda clark.com

The syncrometer and zappicator reduce chemical input. They can be used on pets, food and on our bodies to remove many parasites, eggs and stages of hatching, along with nasty chemicals. Kill the pathogens and clean the blood naturally.

Stop your body becoming a host to these immune system bashing creatures...knock them on the head with simple electronic devices.

www.zappertek.com

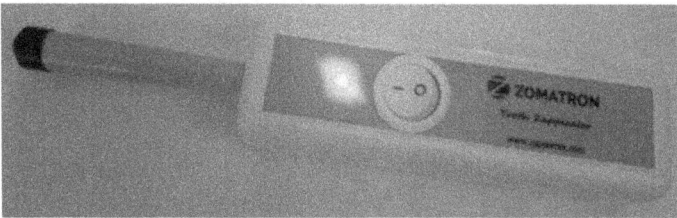

This is a tooth zappicator that reduces the amount of bacteria and parasites in your mouth and teeth, each tooth corresponds to an organ, leaking toxins into the bloodstream, causing disease...

CHAPTER 28

Parasitic Infections.

Here are some horror stories concerning parasites.

1. An 11 month old baby is infected with Baylisascaris procyonis worms that cause him to sleep excessively, lose his balance and is nearly blinded. An elderly war veteran has his legs rendered useless by Lymphatic filariasis caused by Wuchereria bancrofti worms. Doctors discover that a young man has Schistosoma mansoni flukes in his brain, causing nausea and dizziness.

2. A group of teenage students visiting Jamaica are infected with Angiostrongylus cantonensis worms after they ate a contaminated salad. An outbreak of Cryptosporidium hominis occurs in Eastern Wisconsin and kills over a hundred people. Human feces had contaminated the city's water system and the cysts survived despite chlorine treatment.

3. Botfly maggots invade the head of a young man as he travels abroad. A factory worker contracts the Paragonimus kellicotti fluke from eating raw crayfish, causing him to cough up blood. A young woman unknowingly transports bed bugs in her suitcase and into her home from a stay at a hotel.

4. A young girl nearly loses her sight when she contracts Acanthamoeba keratitis from wearing expired contact lenses. An elderly man is infected with Strongyloides stercoralis worms that remained dormant inside his body for over fifty years.

5. A boy nearly loses his sight in one eye due to Toxocara canis. A man is infected with human African trypanosomiasis. A child dies from amoebic meningitis.

6. A woman is infected with Taenia solium cysts that severely weaken the function of her spinal cord. A boy comes down with toxoplasmosis and almost goes blind. A man in the Eastern United States is stricken with malaria.

7. A young dancer's life is put on hold by severe abdominal pain and vomiting. She is found to have decaying Anisakis simplex worms in her colon, most likely caused by eating sushi. A middle-aged man travels to Haiti and has seizures caused by Taenia solium.

8. *A man's liver is nearly destroyed by Entamoeba histolytica. A girl's body is invaded by a parasitic worm called Trichinella spiralis, which causes a red, lumpy rash. A man's stay in an unsanitary hospital ends with a case of scabies.*

9. *A young boy is struck with an Acanthamoeba brain infection which puts him in a coma. A man has extreme Plasmodium falciparum malaria and has post-malarial neurological symptoms two weeks after doctors thought he had recovered. A man contracts leishmaniasis, which destroys his spleen.*

10. *A child suffers from severe vomiting and diarrhea caused by Cryptosporidium contaminated water. A man, who had contracted AIDS, dies from a deadly amoeba known as Balamuthia mandrillaris. A young girl loses sight in one eye due to the invasion of her body by Taenia crassiceps, a rare and particularly nasty tapeworm. She failed to wash her hands after gardening.*

11. *A student travels to South America and contracts leishmaniasis. This was determined after he noticed a mysterious wound that began to grow and ooze. A girl gets a hookworm after being scratched by a kitten. A couple notice a strange rash that appears, then goes away, then appears again. It was caused by the Gnathostoma roundworm they got while on a trip to Africa.*

12. *A woman develops a rash on her groin and upper thighs caused by Schistosoma mansoni, which later causes bladder cancer. A man suddenly has a huge appetite, unusual weight loss, and abdominal pain that turns out to be Ascaris lumbricoides, which was apparently caused by eating contaminated food.*

CHAPTER 29

Gluten and Lectin Intolerance

Both gluten and lectins can contribute to abdominal pain and digestive discomfort, sluggishness, general slowing down of your bodily functions...Leaky gut, brain fog, ADHD in both kids and adults, depression and anxiety and general illness such as celiac disease, rheumatoid arthritis and auto-immune disease.

Lectins don't want to digest, whereas gluten digests through the system but leaves toxins for the body to sort out within its own elimination process in people that have sensitivity to them.

Some examples of lectins are beans, grains and cereals, tomatoes, potatoes, sweet potatoes, mushrooms...some examples of gluten are anything that has wheat flour...pasta, noodles, breads and pastries, crackers, cereals, coating mixes, croutons, flour tortillas, sauces and gravy, beer and brewer's yeast

CHAPTER 30

Dangers of Tap water and fluoride

Fluoride is in tap water which is classified as a waste product from Aluminium and uranium processing. Ingestion has been known to cause brittle teeth and bone disease, discoloured teeth, cancer, heart disease, arthritis and premature aging and have a damaging effect on the pineal gland in the brain.

Chlorine, which is known to contribute to diabetes, cancers, kidney stones and heart attacks, even with the process being cleaned, it seems a good idea to filter all water, even bath water, as this enters the bloodstream via osmosis..

Hitler was known to use it during WW2 to brainwash the prisoners of war.

CHAPTER 31

E-cigs

Electronic cigarettes are marketed as being the healthy alternative to smoking and to help in the "giving up" process... they are in fact, full of bad chemicals, far worse than the original cigarette, if that's possible, and can cause a worse addiction/craving through them.

Nicotine causes heart, brain and nervous system problems, affects the lungs and skin, and causes blood clots and stomach ulcers... Nicotine even from 'quitting' patches or through 'Vaping' can have the same effects.

Diacetyl is added to smokeless cigarettes and can cause an irreversible disease called popcorn lung.

Some smokeless cigarettes have 3-4 times the amount of nicotine than ordinary cigarettes*.

*As at the time of this 2nd edition edit (May/June 2020) the EU has now banned the sale of Menthol cigarettes on the basis that they are perceived as a healthier alternative due to the flavour. Menthol does in fact increase the dilating effect on the pulmonary alveoli causing faster absorption of nicotine.

CHAPTER 32

Microwave pollution

Microwaving deprives your food of most of its nutrients, affects the constitution of the food, leaving it virtually non-nutritious. Microwaves produce benzopyrenes which are carcinogenic, lower the immune system and encourage parasite growth.

Even standing close to your microwave damages you too, exposing you to an electro-magnetic field and radiation; this weakens your defenses and allows cells to grow irregularly, causing disease.

CHAPTER 33

Toxic Colours - Colourings found in foods and clothings.

Kids, Birthday party foods and food colouring.

Kids birthday parties can contain many hidden dangers... apart from making the kids temporarily hyper, there are potentially more serious implications and effects on the body, Found in birthday cakes and cup-cakes, lollipops, candies and jellies.

Blue dye - linked to cancer

Red dye- linked to thyroid tumors

Green dye- linked to bladder cancer

Yellow dye- linked to kidney tumors and adrenal glands

These are used readily in most processed, prepared and packaged foods, Pop/soda, anything coloured has these chemicals in them.

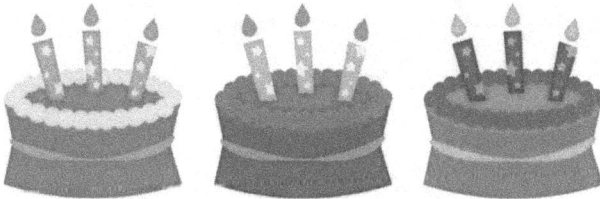

Toxic clothing

After clothes are made, they are often covered with formaldehyde which has been linked to cancer, to keep them from wrinkling or becoming mildewed during shipping.

A number of textile workers have developed severe skin conditions due to their frequent exposure to formaldehyde.

It is recommended that you always wash your new clothes before wearing them, or clothes from thrift stores too get sprayed with chemicals to make them look, and smell better.

Have you ever noticed how undertakers look dead themselves? It must be all that formaldehyde?

Black clothing and dyes for leathers often contains PPD, which can produce allergic reactions. Carcinogenic flame retardants can appear in bedding and nightwear.

Volatile organic compounds (VOCs) and dioxin-producing bleach are used by textile industries, where the materials for clothing are produced. Dioxin, a known carcinogen, absorbed through the skin from clothes, highly toxic and linked to diabetes.

CHAPTER 34

What causes acidity?

The reason acidosis is more common in our society is mostly due to the typical western diet, which is too high in fructose, sugar and wheat, and too low in alkaline-producing foods like fresh vegetables.

We eat acid-producing processed foods and drink acid-producing beverages like coffee and soft drinks. We use too many drugs, reach out for a Tylenol/paracetamol when you get a headache, cough medicine, throat pastilles etc. etc. which are all acid-forming. We use artificial chemical sweeteners which are extremely acid-forming, like NutraSweet, Equal, or aspartame .This in turn causes the body to change from a healthy alkali state to one that invites disease...Acidic!!!

CHAPTER 35

MSG- monosodium glutamate

Causes hormonal imbalances, brain damage, obesity, headaches, severe thirst and dehydration.

Found in processed, prepared and packaged foods...disguised sometimes under different names...also found in Asian and Chinese foods.

Found in bottled sauces, protein powder, salad dressings, vaccines, baby food, salad croutons, spice mixtures, soup, instant formula and soy "meat products.

Anything with glutamate/glutamine (read labels) is carcinogenic and fuels disease.

CHAPTER 36

Toxic weather

Ozone layer- thunderstorms and pollution

In summertime the emissions from the wildfires, fumes from factories and cars, airplanes, burning plastics etc. When these chemicals get into the atmosphere, they can affect the whole earth influencing severe weather changes, tsunamis, hurricanes, tornados.

Chemicals pollute the ozone layer that affect the low and high pressure, heating up the ocean which in turn creates low pressure and escalates the effects of a storm to severe.

Acid rain is the result of chemicals in the atmosphere...

Watch what you put down your drain and toilet, what you burn, what you spray on your garden, these pollutants go into the ground, mix with the water systems in rivers and flow out to sea, and pollute our own gardens, wildlife on the way, whatever you flush down the toilet, bleach, cleaners etc. goes into the grass from the drain, the deer, rabbits, birds eat the grass and the produce from the ground...it also goes into the air... the chemicals from the cleaners, air fresheners and incense, scented candles.

We swim in the seas that have been polluted by these chemicals and microbial bacteria/parasites from lakes and rivers they enter the body, causing mega harm internally and externally, plus the damage done to marine life... the fish you love to eat from the sea and rivers. Use castile soap for dishes, magnets for washing clothes, vinegar and hot water for cleaning (good for mirrors) and essential oils, diluted with water for air freshener.

CHAPTER 37

Toxic home

Are you obsessed with cleaning and germs?

Do you use products to clean and to freshen the house like bleach, anti-bacterial wipes, sprays, air freshener for that "clean" smell.

THINK AGAIN... how many chemicals are you bringing to your home? What are you, your children and pets ingesting?

Most cleaning products contain highly toxic chlorine and fluorine, glycol, halogens, kerosene which affect the brain and central nervous system which cause confusion, mental retardation and headaches... Not only are you damaging the children and pets in the household but Mother Earth too, by putting it all down the drain, onto the ground outside, filling up rivers and harming wildlife, trees.

Flooring and carpets contain benzene, formaldehyde and styrene which are all known carcinogens, the shower curtain and kids toys contain harmful chemicals...such as plasticizers, phthalates, pesticides and asbestos, lead and dioxins.

Non-stick pans are deadly to domestic birds, so imagine what they do to us and more so, to our children and other pets.

Same thing in your car...do you have a nice smelling pine tree stuck to your dashboard... something similar? Do you clean your dashboard with nice smelling wipes that are completely TOXIC?

Any fragrance you smell is automatically polluting your whole system. Indoor air pollution is caused by carpet chemicals, these products cause many problems including: eye, nose, lungs, headaches, nausea, coughing and fatigue. Fragrances have up to 3000 chemicals which are used in perfumes, colognes and deodorants, scented candles, incense, detergents and fabric softeners, dryer sheets...all contributing to allergies and asthma problems too.

How to freshen your home? It sounds simple... open the window.... use essential oils and vinegar, baking soda... STOP POLLUTION.... Keep plants in each room to absorb toxins and increase oxygen levels...

Use a humidifier...put moisture into the room; use only good, clean filtered water to clear the air.

There are many alternatives that we look at in part 2 Toxic Remedies...

CHAPTER 38

Toxic TV

With all the media we hear every day via the television, news and radio. The shootings, crime, aggression, killings, murders, jail sentences. We have movies, newspapers and TV that give people ideas of nastiness and cruelty, especially within this toxic world. They affect people's brains and invite them to copy their actions; violence begets violence the world over.

Churches, sects, religions are all being affected. If people were not given these awful ideas put forward by best-selling number 1 movies then, highly likely, the bad things wouldn't happen. These create negativity which people thrive on, they love disaster and doom, if everyone just thought nice thoughts for a while, the world would be a much better place.

CHAPTER 39

Highest food risks

Smoking is the highest cause of cancer and heart disease but we are subjected to processed foods, barbecued, burnt foods that are causing as much harm and damage to the body as the smoking does without knowing.

Burnt/charred foods contain benzopyrenes which are carcinogenic, lowering the immune system and encouraging parasitic growth.

Foods such as processed meats, baloney, sausages, deli meats, hot dogs, chips, cookies, tinned and frozen vegetables, white bread ...Ready to eat microwave meals, coffee, pop and milk, anything with white refined flour and a shelf life, contains preservatives and chemicals which are carcinogenic, bacon and sausages are one of the main colo-rectal cancer causes, high in nitrites, nitrates and salt /sodium which literally bungs up the system.

High saturated fats plus hormones and antibiotics, with chemical preservatives contribute to cancer. Meat takes three days to pass through the digestive system, putting a lot of pressure on the other organs to process it, causing other illnesses.

Omega 6 - Vegetable oils, canola oils...all fuel for cancer and disease.

Tinned food - The metal in the can goes into the food – then into your system...Acidic foods like fruits in a tin can break down the metal and tuna will absorb toxins from the can, eat fresh wherever possible.

Cheese - A fermented milk product that slows down the systems by taking three days to go through the process and contributes to yeast overgrowth. Dairy products are mucus forming which causes nasal, sinus, skin problems and allergies.

Caffeine- Tea, coffee and pop, wreaks havoc with blood sugar levels and forces your adrenal glands to overwork. These glands get worn out and keep asking for more caffeine, hence the "jitters" you get on caffeine withdrawal causing stress and increasing the cravings for carbs, fats and proteins.

Pop/soda- as with deli foods and sausages etc. pop has been shown to cause cancer with its sugar content, food chemicals and colourings, especially the caramel colour of most colas makes the body acidic and feeds cancer cells.

Popcorn- the bags that are used to microwave popcorn are lined with carcinogenic material which are linked with causing liver, testicular and pancreatic cancers, coupled with the radiation from the microwave you are heading downhill fast.

Fried foods- comfort food that does horrendous things to the body, frying produces molecules that damage the body, "free radicals" – that go round the body attacking cells, causing cancer, premature aging , deep wrinkles, constipation and diarrhea, the two are closely connected, when one blockage is removed you get a blast of diarrhea.

Pasta - did you know pasta and bread contain sugar too?

Simple carbs- soda, candy, sugar, honey, white rice, bread and pasta, the toxins from the wheat and sugar enter the bloodstream, creating allergies that cause headaches, indigestion, fatigue, bad skin and depression.

Too much yeast will cause Candida, infections and yeast overgrowth.

Complex carbs- the healthy options that contain nutrients and vitamins/minerals are brown rice, quinoa, potatoes, beans, peas and lentils...

It has been shown that refined white flour with its high glycemic rate also raises blood sugar levels, along with the carbs that directly feeds cancer cell growth.

These foods and toxins make the whole body acidic, which in turn makes cells attack the weak spots of the body and the healthy ones too...

By using these toxic ingredients the hospitals are kept busy, doctors surgeries filled... Do you want to become another number in the statistics???

We look at healthy options in part 3...So what can we eat?

What this book is saying is everyone has an option, you don't have to throw things away, you don't have to give everything up, but it's better knowing about it and recognizing the straw that breaks the camel's back.

Think about your children and your pets, even if you don't worry about your own health, just by making a few changes you can stop them suffering unnecessarily.

Asthma and allergies build up from birth with diapers (dioxin), baby bath and shampoos, talcum, wipes, exposure to cleaning products.

"MUST have the place clean for the baby"...

Better to use hot water and vinegar, essential oils diluted in a spray bottle.

So things may not smell so good but disease is reduced by half... or more.

Everything in life is a choice...

CHAPTER 40

Toxic mind and thoughts

State of mind

Probably the most important part of your well-being is the mind, how you think and feel about things, people, your job, friends and family, how you are accepted in society, how you see yourself- your appearance.

Spring clean your mind with good thoughts and forgiveness.

Power is toxic unless used wisely and cautiously.

Bitterness, unforgiving, bad thoughts, jealousy and negative emotions and feelings contribute to illness, stress and ill health, both mentally and physically.

Everyone goes through a transitional period in their lives, for various reasons, this teaches you how to deal with these periods.

This creates inspiration amongst those who feel lost, need guidance, to show them another way.

Emotions create good or bad energy.

When you surround yourself with good energy, great things happen, knock on effect, it is amazing...good thoughts bring great happenings...

When you have bad energy around you, things just go wrong, just can't seem to stop the silly annoying things happening, you trip over, have your three bad luck things in a day, type of energy...by using the good energies below and not using the bad energy, you can turn your life around to being totally positive and see results immediately, in all aspects of your life, physically and mentally.

Negative emotions are jealousy, regret, anger, doubt, fear, panic, dread, rage, disgust, sorrow, boredom, frustration, lying, sarcasm, selfishness.

Positive emotions and feelings are happiness, joy, laughing, smiling, singing, and feeling satisfied, pleasure, desire, admiration, triumph, amusement, hope, peacefulness, LOVE, kindness

Gratitude is a very powerful positive emotion, be thankful, you will attract more.

The mind is a powerful thing and capable of much, make sure you look after it and treat it with utmost respect, watch the sugar and chemical load you put on it that cause depression, dementia, anger issues, and ultimately illness and disease within the body, the body and mind are very closely linked.

Reiki can help tremendously with the state of the mind, Qigong, yoga, meditation, exercise- changing your thought pattern, not watching bad movies, T V drama, reading media, it's all negative and transfers to your own thoughts. Don't mix with negative people; they will bring you down to their level.

Fasting can help with your negative emotions and poor state of mind, clearing your mind so you can see the light at the end of the tunnel, part fasting is fine too, according to the Bible.

EVERYTHING REQUIRES EFFORT

CHAPTER 41

Prevention is better than cure

Cancer and disease cannot live in a healthy, oxygen filled body, use magnets to keep a strong magnetic/ionised force, drink essiac tea, use spices such as curcumin, turmeric, juice wheatgrass, juice all veg, use devil's apple, eat red grapes and citrus fruits, all the colours of the rainbow in fresh healthy fruits and vegetables, substitute the man-made processed sugars for fruit like figs and mulberry or pure stevia, drink pure water, use essential oils, in the bath, diffuser, sprays keep nasties at bay and can actually help reduce the symptoms of illness, stick with low glycemic index GI for better health.

Wash your hands after using the PC, tablet or phone especially if using the phone in the kitchen before preparing food, as they harbor bacteria and other pathogens.

Remove the metal fillings from your mouth that are leaching heavy metals into the body. Fix any broken teeth and infections immediately, these correspond to the parts of the body that leak toxins and chemicals into them and the bloodstream, causing diseased organs.

Stay away from GMO corn and wheat especially Glutamate, anything that says glutamate, monosodium we know as MSG which is also linked to cancer. Soy is high in glutamine which is fuel and fertilizer for illness and disease. Sugars, which impair the immune system, attack the brain function and also fuel cancer cells.

Exercise- it cleans the body through increasing oxygen circulation to the blood.

Avoid anything in a packet or a tin.

Take the reins of your own life, be a pioneer, don't end up like this guy here and become a statistic

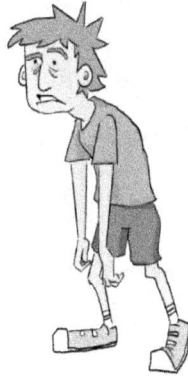

PART 2- TOXIC REMEDIES

Part 2 is to show you the easiest proven way of getting rid of the nasties that have invaded our bodies, by diet, certain foods that detox and some that kill parasites, aids in dieting, toning and becoming super healthy..

Even my daughter was a bit bemused when I said, well; you know toilet roll is toxic too? "Oh no Mummy, what will I wipe my bum with now????"a huge dilemma for a 5 year old!

What I'm trying to do, is make you aware that this is the straw that broke the camel's back, there are so many toxins in our daily lives that we have not a clue about, so by exposing them gently, you can decide which ones you want to keep using, reduce or eliminate altogether ...it's all about choices... no fixed rules.

Healing is automatic when you clean out the body

Chapters - Part 2

Some great remedies and tricks to be fit and well...

CHAPTER 1

Abide by the laws of Mother nature

Don't wait until you are ill before becoming healthy

1) "Never break your fast" i.e.: breakfast- with a heavy meal, light fresh fruit at the most, the body will be sluggish after eating a large breakfast and need to rest.

2) Eat the main meal from midday to 4pm, smaller portions, try not to eat after 6 -7 pm, keep an active mind, most people eat from boredom and habit.

3) Drink distilled or pure filtered water- you will detoxify when you have this which is a good thing, A feeling of 'it made me ill' may happen (short lived detox) but keep going and you will reap the benefits.

4) Add mother tincture apple cider vinegar to your water, sweetened with stevia extract to give mineral boost and aid toxic elimination.

5) Always be determined and strong - know your goals. They are your own- no-one else's - only YOU can do it

6) Cut out sugar and salt- hidden ones from packets too (pop, chips, canned food, microwave food etc.) use stevia and kelp as substitutes. Watch out for HIGH FRUCTOSE CORN SYRUP...DANGER!!!

7) Use all natural personal care products, soaps, creams, perfumes, toothpaste, shampoo, sunscreen etc.

8) Breathe deeply, fresh air...calms and detoxifies...

9) Gentle regular exercise, walking, swimming etc. Increase the oxygen in the body which in turn gradually heals parts of the body.

10) Eat as much raw/organic as possible

11) There is no one pill you can take - the only way is to stop being acidic and toxic. Allow your body to function again, reversing the illness and signs of aging.

12) Juice as much as possible, it will oxygenate your body and cells, making you energized and healthy.

13) Come out of your comfort zone and take a step forward to become healthier.

CHAPTER 2

How to reverse acidity

Acidity versus alkali…

Disease can only live in an acidic body so by eating processed meats, dairy products, drinking alcohol and soda pop, for example, you are turning your body more acidic daily, then the antacids, over the counter meds, make it worse, short term they help, long term they cause havoc with dyspepsia, acid reflux, these are names for a toxic body retaliating against the foods and stuff you have consumed.

Detox by fasting or refraining from consuming sugar, salt and fatty foods, juice fresh vegetables and fruit that have been washed thoroughly, to neutralize acidity, energize and oxygenate the body.

Drink pure magnetized/ionized water to flush through the toxins. Juice as much as possible, this will give your blood oxygen and reduce acidity, there are some yummy recipes at the end of the book…ENJOY!!

Virus in Latin means poison

CHAPTER 3

Health and fitness plan

How to rid yourself of unwanted fat and toxins? get fit and healthy.

Fast one day a week, gradually detox from caffeine (tea, coffee, cola) for an easier cleanse, milk too, tobacco and nicotine. Where possible reduce alcohol and sugar. The more stuff you can detox from before you fast, the easier the clean out will be, and more beneficial to dig down deeper for nasty heavy metals, chemicals and parasites. When fasting do not worry if you don't have any bowel movements, but you may do on and off for the first few days, after your detox expect to have normal 2-3 a day movements when the colon and intestines are unblocked.

This once a week, day fast will shed pounds and pounds however don't be caught up with toxic-hunger. It is a mind over matter issue when your body plays tricks on you. Having to stop detoxing when you eat something to quell a fake hunger pang, that isn't one really, just feels like it, this is a craving which the parasites are causing. Give me sugar... NOW, in the form of pasta, potato chips, chocolate, candy, cakes...the more sugar and salt the better...crave, crave, crave.

You have certain worms craving/feeding off the lactose in the milk and certain ones feeding off the salt, so just remember when you crave, you might want to change your ideas, do some more exercise or read a book rather than feed the unwanted guests inside you!!!

The longer you fast for, the better the result will be but be careful not to overdo it. Any longer than three days, get someone to supervise your condition. You may feel weak, you may be nauseous, or you may feel fabulous.

Exercise, gently at first, up to an hour walking a day, with gentle toning of arms and legs, weights...lots of reps, low weights ... heavy weights, short reps for building muscle...rowing machine for all over workout, ab-crunches, great to create the 6-pack and trim excess fat....shaker weight is great for toning arms and chest too, stretching and torso turning for love-handles and cellulite appearing on legs, unsightly.

Diatomaceous Earth will detox heavy metals from your system; take 1 teaspoon in an 8oz glass of pure water per day for 90 days. Check with your physician before using.

Psyllium husks can help fill you up and provide necessary fibre whilst losing weight and getting fit...

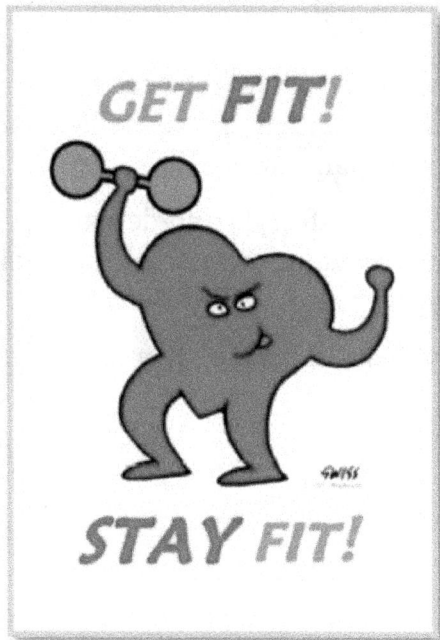

Supplement your diet with vitamin C, E, Magnesium, B complex and Apple cider vinegar for potassium, amino acids and all other minerals that can be lost during exercise, sweating and dieting/ fasting.

Drink copious amounts of water to combat cellulite, provide detox assistance and for its anti-aging properties. Water flushes out toxins from everywhere, skin included. Eat a varied diet of raw veggies and fruit, all washed in filtered water. Cut out sugar and salt, high sodium makes you dehydrated, Pepsi soda being one of the worst culprits.

Sauna and steam baths are great for detoxing. The nasties all come out through the sweat/vapour. Sunshine brings them out too, and adds a valuable source of vitamin D to your body.

Please note that when detoxing, use room temperature drinks, cold water will stop the toxins from passing through the system, holding onto the toxic waste whilst creating flu like symptoms that are quite unpleasant.

Whilst fasting, some people might need to take vitamin B12 to combat the deficiency which can cause light-headedness, that wobbly feeling, heart palpitations.

Maintaining your diet, lifestyle and detoxing regularly, getting quality sleep and reducing stress will all help you become healthier in body and mind.

Don't wait until you are ill before becoming healthy.

CHAPTER 4

Stem Cell Patch Therapy

In the body, there are base stem cells that divide into specialized stem cells for each organ, such as liver stem cells or heart stem cells. This therapy activates these stem cells in each organ, helping to repair and rejuvenate them so they function at their optimum level. Over time, these stem cells can become dormant and impaired, leading to gradual decline and disease. The therapy resets damaged stem cells to a younger, healthier state, improving and repairing other cells in the body, reducing illness and pain.

The therapy uses the body's own copper peptide and stimulates the skin with photo regeneration. It includes patches and treatments for chronic pain, such as muscular problems, joint issues like arthritis, and neuropathy. There are also patches for acute pain, like broken bones and pulled tendons.

The body heat activates patches containing amino acids, oxygen, water, and salts, which then reflect light to activate the stem cells. The brain then signals the body's cells to repair specific areas. This promotes age reversal by increasing biochemicals in the body, supporting wound healing, pain relief, and detoxification. This leads to faster healing, better recovery, and an overall improvement in well-being. The main stem cells in the body are activated, dividing into cells for organs like the liver, heart, and brain, enhancing their function and health.

This therapy also helps with mental illnesses such as Alzheimer's and dementia, which result from damaged cells not functioning properly. By rejuvenating these cells, the therapy can improve cognitive function and slow the progression of these diseases.

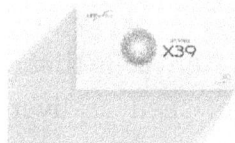

Check out our Website to find out the amazing benefits of using Stem Cell activation patches here: https://www.lifewave.com/631435570

CHAPTER 5

Alternative Methods

ACV - apple cider vinegar, hair conditioner, ringworm killer, cures many skin problems, bug bites, acne, face toner (diluted), deodorant.

Baking soda and sugar - Mixed together in a bowl ...rats eat it and die.

Baking soda - Scouring agent, bath cleaner, sink cleaner, oven cleaner...make a paste with baking soda.

Bath salts - Put apple cider vinegar for skin softening or rashes.

Bites- Bicarbonate of soda for relaxed muscles, to soften the water, and your skin too, Epsom salts will also relax your muscles and detox you, try also using coconut oil added to warm bath this will soothe you and moisturize your skin. *Take care when getting out of the bath as it will be slippery*

Borax - For cockroaches, ants, pests, laundry stains, rust, cleaning the sink, unblocking drains, general bathroom cleaner, floors, toilet, sink cleaner, kills mold (1 cup to a gallon of water, wipe and leave on) disinfects and deodorizes, kills ants.

Carpet deodorizer-Baking soda or a spray of white vinegar.

Castile soap and washing soda - dish detergent/laundry detergent...Borax for heavily stained clothing.

Cooking oil - Coconut oil or olive oil, replace vegetable/canola oil with these.

Cornstarch - Deodorizes, mix with water to form a paste to clean grease.

Essential oils air-freshener – Pick the essential oil of your choice mixed with water use in a BPA free spray bottle.

Essential oils Vacuum cleaner freshener – A cotton wall ball soaked in essential oil of your choice to eliminate pet odors and nasty carpet smells.

Himalayan salt instead of iodized salt, for mineral content.

Lemon juice - Natural disinfectant and bleaching agent. Good for lightening hair in the sun and bleaching dark spots on your skin.

Magnetic Insoles can be used for diabetic nerve pain, to provide energy for sports people and relief for people with joint pain or discomfort.

Magnets for laundry. A set of strong magnets in your washing machine, no detergent, washes clean and no rinse needed, it saves on detergent and water, and comes out softer than using a conditioner. For extra stains use grated natural soap or Castile soap rubbed into stain, when washing clothes that have solvents from external sources and other chemicals from the workplace, wash them separately from your children's clothes, or you risk contaminating their clothes too.

The same goes for your pet's bedding. You don't want solvents, pesticides, plasticizers and heavy metals transferred to your pet either.

Peppermint essential oil and water mix - 20 drops to a litre spray bottle for mice deterrent, spider deterrent and bug repellent, Citronella/lemongrass oil works well too.

Plant insecticide /dish detergent - Castile soap with water mixed, sprayed on leaves, neem oil diluted.

Sugar - use Stevia instead, pure extract or the leaf itself. Most packet-prepared Stevia is mainly cellulose-sawdust.

Substitute perfume, which has 3,000 chemicals in, with pure essential oils of your choice. Mixed with carrier oil, synthetic oils are even more toxic so beware...

Toothpaste - Mix your own with coconut oil, neem oil, essential oils of peppermint, oregano, thyme and cinnamon bark, use baking soda if required.

Vinegar- Natural disinfectant and deodorizer ½ water ½ vinegar mix for grease and mildew

CHAPTER 6

Benefits of Stevia (can help you to stop smoking too)

Stevia is an amazing plant, it actually tastes incredibly sweet. Used for baking, cooking and sweetening without the calories or problems that arise from sugar.

Can also be used for skin problems, added to balms, anti-aging when added to face creams, diabetes relief, gingivitis, heartburn, indigestion, high blood pressure, osteoporosis, weight loss and addiction aid. Stevia helps with stopping smoking and alcohol addiction...it stops the nicotine cravings by blocking the signals from the brain. Try putting some drops on the tongue when you want a cigarette and it will instantly stop the craving.

A wonder plant... We have one growing in our windowsill right now!

Use pure leaves - make a tea and use a few drops of the solution to replace sugar or the packet/liquid forms of sweeteners that you can buy in the supermarket, as they are laced with preservatives, arsenic and other chemicals.

CHAPTER 7

Magnets

Magnetic therapy works by increasing the flow of oxygen through the blood allowing it to reach the parts of the body that are hurt, blocked from normal blood flow, causing disease and pain (must not be used with a pacemaker/hearing aid or any battery operated aid)

Use by gradually increasing the gauss levels, if you are not used to the force, increased blood flow can cause dizziness and nausea as oxygen reaches the weak parts, but unlikely if used under supervision.

Disease cannot live in a strong magnetic force, or highly ionized charge, thereby the ph. level is reduced creating a healthy alkali form. This applies to the earth too, we do our laundry and dishes, bath and shower, using toxins, this all goes out through the drain into the earth, into our water supply, onto our vegetable gardens and fruit trees, the chickens eat and drink the toxic water and food available i.e. grass and seeds, fruits from the trees...the same as our wildlife.

Magnetise the water in your household, you will have "live" water that will benefit everything it touches, turning it into a healthy safe to use product. Bathe in the magnetized water it will eliminate the toxins that you would have absorbed by osmosis and leave you feeling great, you will save on skin softeners. Save laundry detergent by using strong magnets in your washing machine, high gauss level magnets will remove bacteria, mould and dirt from your clothes leaving them undamaged from exposure to chemicals in normal detergents. Magnets can be used in all types of washing machines. It leaves your clothes as soft as if you used a fabric softener (they are also toxic)

Other magnetic products include:

Insoles for neuropathy, diabetic nerve pain relief, joint pain and boosting energy.

Necklace for tonsils, thyroid, thymus, neck, cervical, throat and respiratory conditions.

Eye mask for total relaxation of the brain, eyes, helping short and long sightedness, sinus problems and upper respiratory issues.

Back and belly belt for kidneys, adrenal glands, spinal discomfort, obesity, digestive disorders.

Disease cannot live in a strong magnetic force.

Live magnetic water reduces acidity, helps reduce disease within the body, is great for plants and yields more fruit and veg. It's good for washing fruit and veggies in, animals love it too. It can help reduce any symptoms of illness they may have and make them a healthier pet.

How to make magnetic water?

Take a strong north-pole magnet (see my page on Magnetic Therapy Health - https://www.facebook.com/MagneticTherapyHealth/ select a 2500-3500 gauss level magnet and place it under a water pitcher, glass or BPA free plastic container. Leave for 30 minutes, use as and when you need it, replace after each refill, can be used in humidifiers, face sauna and oil burners...anything you put into the air should be filtered and magnetized , or the chemicals will still cause problems within yours and your pet's body, good via inhalation and osmosis (through the skin).

PEMF / Pulsed Magnetic Therapy -Bio magnetic pulsed therapy treats joints, ligaments, tendons, deep tissue, wounds, post-surgery, depression and anxiety amongst many other conditions.

The machine removes layers of build-up in arteries and veins, blood vessels and nerves as well as accelerating healing to all parts of the body.

Non-invasive, high gauss level treatment that floods your body with oxygen, allowing blood to reach the parts that were originally starved, regenerating and reversing signs of aging and damage.

Illness and disease cannot survive in oxygen.

CHAPTER 8

Superfoods and healing tonics

Almonds (sprouted and dried) are an excellent source of vitamin E and a natural cholesterol reducer.

Aloe Vera leaves contain 20 minerals, 12 vitamins and 18 amino acids. They have excellent digestive healing properties for conditions such as Candida, ulcers, irritable bowel syndrome and inflammation. They are also used topically for wounds, burns and skin problems.

Astragalus is a root that is a good tonic for the immune system. It can enhance the function of the skin to eliminate toxins. Increases white blood cells and can be taken for prolonged periods.

Cacao beans (or powder)...are the raw beans from which chocolate is made. The bean is very nutritious and has a large amount of antioxidants and amino acids. They are a good source of magnesium helping build bones and a healthy heart. It is often called "nature's Prozac"due to its serotonin, dopamine and phenylethylamina content, known neuro-transmitters which help relieve depression.

Chia Seeds are high in omega 3, have anti-inflammatory effects on joints, and are pain relieving .They contain 20-25% protein. They slow down the absorption of carbohydrates thereby controlling blood sugar levels.

Goji Berry helps support the adrenal gland and kidneys resulting in enhanced stamina, strength, longevity and sexual energy, also boosting the immune system, improving eyesight, increasing alkalinity and vitality, they contain 21 trace elements and 19 amino acids.

He Shou Wu – Used to clean the liver and kidneys. The high zinc content helps with DNA repair and restores damaged cell membranes.

Hemp seeds are a complete protein source, have a high content of the E.F.A omega 3, protein is not only for building muscles, ligaments and tendons but for endurance, balanced blood sugar, detoxification and blood thinning to prevent blood clots. Hemp has 20 trace minerals, 18 amino acids and is 55 % protein.

Maca is a root that has been used for centuries as a tonic and a food to increase stamina and vitality and also to assist hormones caused by bad estrogens from plastic food containers and soy products. It can also relieve symptoms of chronic fatigue.

Reishi Mushroom has traditionally been used as an anti-aging herb and it is considered to be capable of building body resistance, detoxing the body and tissues.. Reishi is believed to prolong life, enhance intelligence and wisdom, also helps regulate blood sugar levels and has powerful anti-tumor properties.

Spirulina has a very high nutrient content being over 60% protein. It has a high concentration of vitamin A (beta-carotene) 10 times more than carrots... it is 1% chlorophyll (one of the highest concentrations in any plant) it cleanses and detoxifies.

Suma powder is good for mental and physical stress, it contains 19 amino acids and germanium, a powerful antioxidant, also iron, cobalt, magnesium and silica..

Zeolite is a mineral for removing heavy metals and toxins from the body. It has a negatively charged molecule that attracts toxins.

CHAPTER 9

Natural person care products

Soaps made with all natural chia seeds, charcoal for detoxing and exfoliation, lime, bergamot and sandalwood essential oils for concentration, and detoxing...

Scrubs...to exfoliate dead cells and leave your skin feeling like silk. Face cream....softens and moisturizes with secret natural ingredients for optimum luxury..

Lip balm enriched with vitamin E for hours of supple lips

Perfume natural essential oils with carrier oil, in a roller ball dispenser

Magnesium oil is easy to apply for irritability and muscle cramps..

Commercial care products

Many commercial care products contain parabens, dioxin, triclosan, sodium lauryl sulfate and phthalates which are all linked to male reproductive, breathing issues, kidney and brain problems, irritated skin, eye problems, organ developmental problems. These are found in shampoos, nail polish, laundry detergents, toothpaste, deodorants, cosmetics, clothing. Talc is a known carcinogen and contributes to ovarian cancer.

CHAPTER 10

Aromatherapy

This is the practice of using essential oils, either in a diffuser, or carrier oil for massage, in a spray bottle for room freshener...

Aromatherapy has many therapeutic uses, for muscle aches, depression, stimulation, insomnia, relaxation. Some can be used in the bathtub, some applied directly to the skin, but most with carrier oil. Certain essential oils can be very strong and damage skin if undiluted, extremely powerful to combat disease.

Used in natural toothpaste, and to treat diseases with its antibacterial, anti-fungal, antibiotic properties, to fragrance natural perfumes and shampoos, soaps and creams.

Lavender for headaches and skin.

Thyme for spots and bites.

Oregano, antiseptic internally and externally, can expel worms.

Vanilla, often used in perfumes to relax.

Tea tree as an antiseptic, anti fungal.

Sandalwood for concentration and meditation.

Oil of cloves for toothache.

Some oils you shouldn't use whilst pregnant.

Research which oil is right for you.

Create a mood with divine aromas.

CHAPTER 11

Benefits of Turmeric

Turmeric contains curcumin, a substance with powerful anti-inflammatory and antioxidant properties. Turmeric is best combined with black pepper to increase absorption into the bloodstream.

It helps with brain function, heart disease, cancer, Alzheimer's.

Suggested as beneficial for arthritis and depression.

Can be added to smoothies, salads, used in cooking, used as a paste topically and in toothpaste.

CHAPTER 12

Benefits of charcoal

Make sure you use activated charcoal and not the barbecue version. It works by trapping toxins and chemicals in its millions of tiny pores. It detoxes the body by ridding them of these nasties and flushing them out...

Great for whitening teeth, used in toothpastes or alone, for gum disease, oral health in general...good for treating poisonings, alcohol poisoning and food too. Drink lots of water when ingesting it as it can cause dehydration. Used as a compress for bug bites, filters tap water from all its toxins...can be used as an antidote for overdose of many pharmaceutical drugs and over-the-counter medications. It's effective for aspirin, opium, cocaine, morphine and acetaminophen. Reduces gas and bloating and is a good digestive cleanse.

CHAPTER 13

Benefits of Neem oil

Neem oil is antibacterial, anti-parasitic, greatly beneficial for flea and tick treatments on your pets, (bath your dog in it, rub it into the gland areas of your pet)Great for keeping your skin clear, anti-aging, good for cavities, add to toothpaste, works well in creams for mosquito bites along with zinc oxide and thyme or oregano essential oil. Helps psoriasis, acne, dry itchy skin, fights fungal infections such as athlete's foot, ringworm and nail fungus.

Used on plants and gardens in a diluted spray for stopping bug attacks, Mosquito, flea and tick invasion. As a natural pesticide, that does no harm to your crop, children and pets.

CHAPTER 14

Benefits of coconut oil

There are many benefits of coconut oil, from massage oil to baking/cooking, making natural soaps and detergents, face creams, lip balms, scrubs, cosmetics, hair conditioners. Coconut aids the digestive system, weight loss, dental care, Candida, immune system, infections, HIV and cancer, kills bacteria that causes throat infections and ulcers.

Coconut helps in controlling blood sugar, and improves the secretion of insulin. It also promotes the effective use of blood glucose, thereby preventing and treating diabetes.

Coconut oil helps boost energy and endurance, and generally enhances the performance of athletes. Also used for oil pulling in the mouth to rid gums and teeth of bacteria.

CHAPTER 15

Benefits of Black Pepper

Due to its antibacterial properties, pepper is used to preserve food. Black pepper is a very good anti-inflammatory agent.

Black pepper contains the minerals potassium, calcium, magnesium, phosphorus, sodium, as well as vitamins such as thiamin, riboflavin, niacin, and vitamin B6. Pepper contains beneficial nutrients including vitamin E, Folate (a B vitamin), and vitamin K.

Black pepper aids in weight loss, helps in relieving sinus, asthma, and nasal congestion. It also reduces the risk of cancer, and can help heart and liver conditions.

Consuming pepper increases the hydrochloric acid in the stomach, thereby facilitating digestion. Proper digestion is essential to avoid intestinal issues including diarrhea, constipation, and colic.

In Ayurvedic (Indian) medicine, pepper is added to tonics for treating cold and cough. Pepper also provides relief from sinusitis and nasal congestion. It has an expectorant property that helps break up the mucus and phlegm depositions in the respiratory tract. Soups made with black pepper and other aromatic spices are often used to treat colds and coughs.

The antibacterial property of black pepper helps fight against infections and insect bites, it also facilitates the cleaning of arteries.

CHAPTER 16

Benefits of Arginine

This truly is a wonderful amino acid, facilitating the blood flow and circulation to the arteries and vessels, veins and nerves, muscles etc.

It turns into nitric oxide- causing blood vessels to open more- and helps the body build protein improving immune system function, male virility (erectile dysfunction) fertility, detoxification, brain function, heart health, muscle repair and wound healing.

It promotes healthy weight loss by burning off the fat. Arginine Improves athletic performance, prevents hair loss and helps the metabolism of sugar so therefore could be beneficial to diabetics to control the blood glucose level.

Supplements are available. Naturally available in watermelon – the amino acid L-citrulline converts into L-arginine. Also found in meats and liver.

CHAPTER 17

Benefits of Apple Cider Vinegar

Apple cider vinegar ingestion can help acid reflux, lower blood pressure, improve diabetes and support weight loss.

The benefits of apple cider vinegar come from the amino acids and high mineral content which include acetic acid, potassium, probiotics, magnesium and enzymes.

Taken daily as a drink diluted in pure filtered magnetic water with a dash of stevia for its properties and taste, helps digestion, energy levels, leg cramps, cleans the body through particularly tendons and ligaments that get clogged up with acid through excess work, great for before and after gym work to decrease the uric acid build up within the muscles.

ACV curbs appetite, is a natural hair conditioner as a rinse, it leaves hair soft and shiny. It removes stains from your teeth, kills off bacteria, a great detox and balancer of the ph. level of the body.

ACV helps with acid reflux and Candida, a great natural house cleaner, even on mirrors!!!

ACV heals poison ivy, fungal infections, flea/skin treatment as a spray or rinse on your pets, add a little to their drinking water too for optimum health, and skin toner.

ACV breaks up mucus in your body and supports lymphatic drainage, helping allergies. It supports the immune system and can clear your sinuses. Put 2 tablespoons in a large glass of water and drink three times daily for allergies.

Used as a natural deodorant, kills off bacteria and cleans pores under the arms.

CHAPTER 18

Diatomaceous earth

In our home you will always find a large tub of Diatomaceous earth (DE)

We use DE every day that we are detoxing and for our pets too.

DE is a naturally occurring sedimentary rock that is composed of the fossilized remains of diatoms, a type of hard-shelled algae. It is typically found in deposits near bodies of water such as rivers, lakes, and oceans. DE is primarily composed of silica, a mineral that is essential for various bodily functions.

In its powdered form, diatomaceous earth is often used for a variety of health purposes. Some of its **potential benefits** include:

1. Detoxification: Diatomaceous earth is believed to have detoxifying properties due to its ability to absorb heavy metals and toxins in the digestive tract, helping to eliminate them from the body.

2. Digestive health: DE may promote digestive health by gently scrubbing the digestive tract, aiding in the removal of waste and promoting regular bowel movements.

3. Joint and bone health: The silica content in diatomaceous earth is thought to support healthy bones and joints by promoting the absorption of calcium and other minerals essential for bone strength.

4. Skin and hair health: Some people use diatomaceous earth topically as a gentle exfoliant to remove dead skin cells and

impurities, promoting smoother, healthier skin. It may also be used in hair care products to help remove product buildup and improve scalp health.

5. Pest control: In addition to its health benefits, diatomaceous earth is also commonly used as a natural pesticide and insecticide. Its abrasive texture can help to effectively kill insects by damaging their exoskeletons, making it a popular choice for controlling pests in gardens and homes.

It's important to note that while diatomaceous earth is generally considered safe for consumption and topical use, it's always best to consult with a healthcare professional before using it for health purposes, especially if you have any underlying health conditions or concerns. Additionally, not all diatomaceous earth products are food-grade, so it's essential to ensure that you are using a high-quality, food-grade product if you intend to consume it.

CHAPTER 19

Magnesium oil/Magnesium and potassium

Magnesium oil is made from Magnesium chloride flakes and sprayed onto your wrists, for a magnesium boost to those that need it (as a spray it can cause irritation and tingling, if this occurs, dilute with pure water) Good for brittle bones, low energy levels, anxiety, irritability, weakness, insomnia, hormonal problems, nervousness, headaches and heart palpitations.

Can be added to the bath as bath salts, makes for a nice relaxing time, a just before bedtime treat. Available in supplement, effervescent and pill form. This works very well when combined with potassium for cleansing the liver. Helping to stave off cravings, assisting blood sugar level control and detoxifying the body.

CHAPTER 20

Benefits of wheatgrass

What does a racehorse eat? Grass… and wins races.

High chlorophyll, grass is beneficial for so many things

Aids digestion taken as a juice.

As a rinse it's good for graying hair and dandruff.

Add it to the bath for psoriasis and eczema.

Use its antiseptic properties to heal cuts and bites, poison ivy and Athlete's foot.

Reduces food cravings and regulates blood sugar levels.

Anti-inflammatory properties, helps to relieve arthritis and sinus inflammation,

It cleans the blood and detoxes the body, including the liver.

Wheat grass can be used as an enema with great success, so many health benefits.

As always… Avoid using it if you are allergic to wheat!

CHAPTER 21

Parasite/Toxin Cleanse

No-one can live in a bubble and be totally protected from these environmental chemicals and parasites so we do what we can, knowing there are toxins in everything we generally use, so take note and beware, use as many natural products as possible.

Fast where possible, even an extended day is good. Give your body a break to rid itself of all the nasties. Zap where possible, do Candida cleanses, liver and kidney cleanses, eat as much organic food as you can.

There are several different forms of what causes illness, bacteria, virus (meaning poison in Latin) stones, cancers, tumors, infection, chemicals/toxins, these can be zapped away, then travel out of the body through the skin, bowels, urinary tract.

The average diet never allows the body to cleanse itself. We eat all the time. When intake of calories is greater than burned, the results will be stored body fat...simple but true. It is the same with toxins. When intake of toxins is greater than removed, the results will be toxic overload. If you are overweight this is a sign you are carrying around a load of toxins, affecting normal bodily functions.

There are many herbs/oils that can be used to expel worms and parasites from the digestive tract such as oil of oregano, wormwood, black-walnut tincture, pumpkin seeds, coconut oil and garlic.

Alternatively use Hulda Clark's 'zapper' for removal, which consists of holding 2 copper rods on the end of a circuit board run by a 9 volt battery, this vibrates at a frequency that will kill off any parasite in your body yet not high enough to harm any organs. Do not use it if you wear a pacemaker.

Diatomaceous Earth will also kill parasites in your system and remove heavy metals, take 1 teaspoon of food grade DE with water every day, on an empty stomach one or two hours after eating. It doesn't taste of anything, so not unpleasant, you reap the rewards in the removal of nasties.

Dental care/toothpaste

By using this formula every day with magnetized water you can reverse oral cavities, keep bacteria and parasites away and have clean whiter teeth by brushing gently twice a day.

Coconut oil ¼ tsp.

Turmeric ¼ tsp.

Clove oil 2 drops

Baking soda – a pinch of

Neem oil ¼ tsp.

Oregano oil 2 drops

Cinnamon bark oil 2 drops

Mix together and keep in a sealed container

CHAPTER 22

Benefits of figs

Due to their high mineral and vitamin content they are a valuable super-food and have been known to...

- Increase energy
- Kill bacteria, roundworm and virus in the body
- Applied directly to a boil/wart can significantly reduce the inflammation
- Softens skin, as a paste
- Promotes hair growth
- Lowers blood pressure
- Provide a great source of fibre helping piles and constipation
- Clears blockages in the liver
- Can help prevent macular degeneration
- Fights sore throats
- Fig juice to relieve asthmatic symptoms
- Helps with erectile dysfunction
- Restores the sodium balance in the body
- Lowers cholesterol
- Enhances digestive function
- Recipe in part 3 for fig cake.

CHAPTER 23

Health benefits of Prickly Pears and Cactus Juice

- Helps osteoporosis
- Boosts immune system
- Reduces risk of cancer
- Reduces risk of heart disease
- Relieves arthritis and gout
- Helps dental care
- Helps weight loss

An alkaline forming fruit, reverses the body's acidity, is very high in vitamin C, has strong anti-inflammatory properties and is full of disease fighting nutrients. Great as a juice, it can cause diarrhea when consumed in large quantities though.

CHAPTER 24

Wild lettuce

Nature has given us plants that can be used to fight sickness, reduce pain, and promote a healthy and balanced life overall.

The leaf, sap and seed of wild lettuce are used to make medicine.

It is used for whooping cough, asthma, urinary tract problems, cough, trouble sleeping (insomnia), restlessness, excitability in children, painful menstrual periods, excessive sex drive in women (nymphomania), muscular or joint pains, poor circulation, swollen genitals in men (priapism), and as an opium substitute in cough preparations.

The seed oil is used for "hardening of the arteries" (atherosclerosis) and as a substitute for wheat germ oil.

The latex can be applied directly to the skin to kill germs. Some people inhale it for a recreational "high" or hallucinogen. It has a calming, relaxing, and pain relieving effect.

CHAPTER 25

Vitamins & Minerals, the benefits

Calcium - Take for muscle cramps, brain function, bone problems and osteoporosis. Overdose can cause kidney stones and calcium deposits in the joints.

Folic acid - Take when preparing to get pregnant and whilst pregnant for the baby's neurological health.

Iron-Take for weakness, fatigue, headaches, cracked lips, difficulty concentrating, brittle nails, Anemia

Magnesium - Take for muscle cramps/spasms, lung and brain function, irritability, anxiety also aids digestion.

Potassium - Take for nausea, muscle weakness, irritability, anorexia, diarrhea...as you lose potassium through bodily functions and sweating...

Sulphur - Detoxifies, cabbage family are prime examples.

Vitamin A - Take for night sight, dry rough skin, dry nose, resistance to infection.

Vitamin B - complex - Take for an energy boost, good for the nervous system, digestive system, concentration and memory.

Vitamin B-12 –A Deficiency can cause weakness, tiredness, light-headedness, and heart-palpitations.

Vitamin C- High dosage can be taken for colds/flu, helps skin, healing of body, rejuvenation of cells and tissues, after stressful situations take Vitamin C to get your body back on track, or take continuously as a preventative measure. Be careful not to take too much as you will experience diarrhea, if your body is unfamiliar to the potency.

Vitamin E- Take for skin problems, hair and nail growth, heals wounds.

You will get 99.9% of your mineral and vitamin needs from a correct diet, only needing to supplement when illness occurs or poor diet.

CHAPTER 25

Spirulina and Chlorella

Spirulina is a microscopic blue-green algae . It is known as a superfood due to its composition and its therapeutic properties.

Spirulina concentrates 20 times more protein than soy and 400 times more than beef. In addition, it is a powerful regenerator of the intestinal microbiota and a powerful activator of cellular detoxification mechanisms.

Its composition is based on a multitude of vitamins, minerals and antioxidants, mainly Vitamins A, B, C, D, E, and K, Potassium, Magnesium, Iodine, Phosphorus, Iron and Sulfur, nucleic acids (DNA and RNA), fatty acids essential nutrients, chlorophyll and an extensive repertoire of phytochemicals with antioxidant effects.

Spirulina is composed of 65% complete plant protein that provides the eight essential amino acids. It is considered an essential microalgae, especially for athletes, because it is very rich in Iron, Potassium and Calcium, and barely contains Sodium. It is also used as an appetite suppressant, making it very useful in weight loss diets. Its richness in chlorophyll makes Spirulina a great blood detoxifier.

The benefits of Spirulina are many thanks to its varied composition. The most notable are:

1. **Non-animal protein source** : Spirulina proteins contain all essential amino acids. Its protein is as complete as that of animal meat and much more complete than that found in plants,

including the proteins provided by legumes. All this makes it a natural alternative to the consumption of animal protein, especially in vegetarian diets.

2. **Antioxidant** : Spirulina contains many vitamins, especially Vitamin A (in the form of Beta-carotene), Vitamin C, Vitamin K and Group B Vitamins. Spirulina is an important source of antioxidant Carotenoids, which once absorbed are transformed into Vitamin A. Carotenoids, Vitamin A and Vitamin C are important cell protectors and antioxidants, essential in the prevention of premature aging and degenerative diseases.

3. **Fights anemia** : Spirulina increases hemoglobin in states of anemia. This circumstance promotes the improvement of blood quality and the increase in the production of red blood cells, given its great richness in iron, its impressive concentration of chlorophyll and its content of phycocyanin, the blue pigment that contributes to inducing the production of cells. mother in the bone marrow.

4. **Strengthens the immune system** : Spirulina increases the production of antibodies and cytokines, which include interferons and interleukins, and improves the state of the immune system, developing great protection against infections, microbes and viruses.

5. **Eliminates heavy metals** : Spirulina, thanks to its powerful antioxidant properties, helps eliminate heavy metals from the body, for example mercury, lead or arsenic, and helps purify and detoxify it, in general.

6. **Inhibits the proliferation of Candida** : In the same way that Spirulina has been proven to strengthen the immune system, it has also been shown to inhibit the proliferation of Candida.

7. **Nourishes hair cells** : Spirulina, thanks to its high protein and mineral content, such as Zinc and Group B Vitamins, nourishes hair cells and helps hair look stronger and shinier. Its essential

fatty acids help improve circulation, preventing its loss. At the same time, it promotes the health of nails and skin.

8. Improves vision : Spirulina has been used to treat Vitamin A deficiencies, responsible for vision loss in people whose diet is deficient in this vitamin.

9. Satiety Effect : Spirulina is very rich in fiber, especially mucilage, which causes satiating effects.

Chlorella is a green, single-celled microscopic algae that grows in fresh waters . Belonging to the Chlorellaceae family and has an important nutritional value, since it contains a high concentration and variety of essential nutrients, especially proteins, vitamins and minerals.

Chlorella is the plant with the highest concentration of chlorophyll. It has between 5 and 10 times more chlorophyll than any other species. It contains almost 60% protein of high biological value.

Thus, its protein content is much higher than that of soy, tuna or beef. It has the growth factor CGF, very rich in nucleic acids, necessary to build, renew, repair and maintain different human organs. It contains a high amount of carotenoids, including high amounts of Vitamin C, Group B Vitamins (including Vitamin B12), Choline and Inositol.

It provides a wide variety of minerals, including Iron, Zinc, Iron, Magnesium, Calcium, Manganese, Copper, Iodine and Cobalt. It stands out mainly for its high content of Iron and Zinc, very important for vegans and vegetarians.

The most notable benefits of Chlorella are:

1. Strengthens the immune system : Its richness in nucleic acids, proteins, vitamins and minerals, stimulates the formation of defensive cells, in addition to the production of red blood cells.

2. **Stimulates growth** : Chlorella's DNA is programmed to quadruple its growth. This is what is known as Chlorella Growth Factor. This property of Chlorella, when ingested as a dietary supplement orally, helps stimulate the growth of children and adolescents. In adults, this growth factor helps repair damaged tissues in the body such as wounds and ulcers, promoting rapid recovery from injuries and diseases, as well as skin regeneration, which means that the cellular aging process is slowed down. slows down.

3. **Protects against free radicals** : The richness of Chlorella in Vitamin C and D, as well as Chlorophyll and Beta-carotene, guarantee powerful antioxidant protection.

4. **Improves the functioning of the digestive system** : Chlorella is rich in fiber, which is why it improves intestinal peristalsis and stimulates the growth of beneficial bacteria for the intestine.

5. **Helps lose weight** : Chlorella also helps lose weight. In fact, the results of several studies have shown that Chlorella helps reduce body fat.

6. **Detoxifies the body** : The Chlorophyll contained in Chlorella is one of the most powerful substances to purify the intestinal microbiota and the lymphatic system, as well as the liver and blood.

CHAPTER 27

Reflexology

To perform Acupressure on both hands and feet, apply pressure on each point shown in the diagram which corresponds to the part of the body indicated to relieve pain, inflammation, discomfort...by using thumbs or fingers , gently push and hold .. Magnetic insoles are good for working all the above points of the body and especially helpful for diabetic nerve problems.

REFLEX ZONES OF THE HANDS

REFLEX ZON

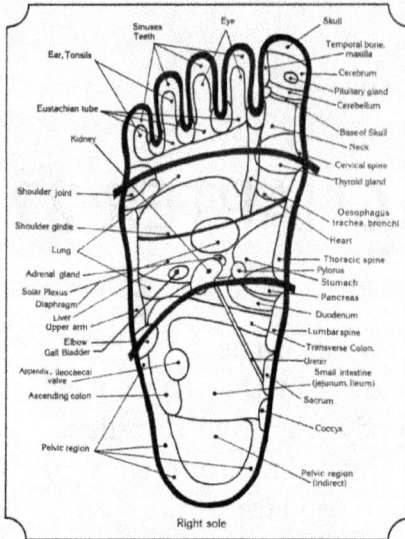

Right sole

S OF THE FEET

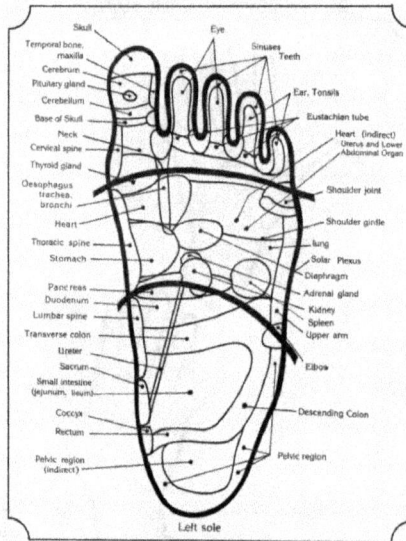

Left sole

Shiatsu/full body massage is also very beneficial using acupressure points and a rolling technique for clearing the body's acid build up

CHAPTER 28

Homeopathy

Homeopathy is a therapy that treats the body as a whole being, It is a natural, safe and gentle medicine. Poison ivy, for example, is treated with Belladonna, which is a poison itself. Arnica treats bruising and accidents, aconite treats shock and after effects of extreme exposure to cold.

Homeopathic remedies come from substances that come from plants, minerals, or animals, such as red onion, arnica (mountain herb), white arsenic, poison ivy, belladonna (deadly nightshade), and stinging nettle. They are often formulated as sugar pellets to be placed under the tongue; they may also be in other forms, such as ointments, gels, drops, creams, and tablets

Remedies come in different doses and different strengths for different illnesses. Non-invasive treatment, very effective with no side effects. With each dilution the dose gets stronger 6c, 30c, 100c. There are 2,500 different remedies.

CHAPTER 29

Chi Kung

A super way to increase your own energy by slow movements designed to increase vitality and health. Pronounced "Qigong" in English, it is the training of your energy to be utilized in the best possible way by doing simple exercises in the quiet of your own home, with nature, or in a class. You gain incredible energy within your whole body which can then be tuned into healing, advancing in spiritual ways, getting in tune with your inner self, keeping fit in body and mind, creating your own amounts of energy to vitalize you and propel you through the day to meet anything in your path.

CHAPTER 30

Castor oil wraps

Using a flannel, sheet of plastic and a heat pad, dip the flannel into the oil, place it on the skin, abdomen area or problem area and leave for 45 minutes, repeat 3 -7 days for detoxing purposes.

Aids: Congestion, liver problems, arthritis, kidney problems, headaches, toxic waste removal, digestive disorders, nervous system and weight loss.

Great topically for skin problems: Acne and spots, under eye bags, great for re-hydrating exhausted skin. Helps by replacing elasticity lost through aging and sun exposure, drawing out unwanted toxins and regenerating the body.

CHAPTER 31

Rescue Remedy and Bach flower remedies

These remedies work on a vibrational level to aid your emotions that stop your body from healing. Rescue remedy can be used on children, pets, horses and adults alike. It is used for shock, as an emergency help, after a fall or disappointment, to be able to cope with life.

A safe and gentle form of healing with no reported side effects.

By using a combination of these therapies you can be assured to have a healthy, happy mind and body.

CHAPTER 32

Harmless/non-toxic versus toxic/bad for you

To recap on some of the previously covered comparisons.

1) Magnets for washing versus normal detergent for dishes and laundry.

2) Magnetic filtered water to drink and wash in versus tap water and BPA plastic bottled water/bath and shower water.

3) Vegetables and fruit washed in magnetized water which removes parasites and pesticides along with the zappicator- see chapter 31 versus tinned veg and fruit - leeched heavy metals and preservatives/E numbers.

4) Coconut oil/olive oil for cooking versus canola oil

5) Natural soap –essential oil perfumed and no chemicals added versus commercial soap with parabens and sodium lauryl sulfate plus many more.

6) Vinegar/H2O2/steamer to clean products versus bleaches and detergents of commercial cleaning.

7) White natural bristled toothbrush versus coloured toothbrushes.

8) Natural toothpaste (see recipes) versus fluoride toothpaste.

9) Natural deodorant, face cream, deodorants, soaps and essential oils versus named products, commercial deodorant, creams, perfumes and soaps.

10) Humidifiers with essential oil scent – if needed (put moisture into the air) versus commercial air fresheners.

11) Essential oil sprays for freshness/beeswax candles versus scented candles, incense and plug in air fresheners.

12) Sterilized cloths and sponges versus kitchen roll and paper towels (both bleached).

13) Filtered, magnetized water for you, your pets and plants versus tap water with chemicals added.

14) Oregano essential oil or thyme oil for cuts or sores, cold/flu symptoms and infection. Antifungal works as an antiseptic and rids mycotoxins versus Neosporin/named brands antiseptic cream and over the counter flu drugs.

CHAPTER 33

Raw Energy

Eating lots of veggies and fruits helps control blood pressure.

The diet is low in sodium, so it can help lower your chance of stroke, heart failure, osteoporosis, stomach cancer, and kidney disease.

Losing weight and keeping it off, can help prevent or manage type 2 diabetes.

Eating mainly raw is so much easier for your digestive tract to pass food through the body, therefore allowing the rest of the organs to do the healing job they need to do, expelling toxins...

They are high in fibre, contain many vitamins and minerals, aid weight loss being low in calories and give you increased energy.

If you fast, exercise, detox regularly and eat a good diet of fresh foods you will never have any reason to take medication, as your body will heal itself, you will be at optimum weight, and have minimal reason for any complaints.

CHAPTER 34

Tongue and signs of toxicity

Tongue scraper- use a tongue scraper to ensure NO bad breath (halitosis)...

Takes away bacteria from the tongue in a few scrapes...

Your tongue is a tell-tale sign of ill health...we know through discolouration and the fuzz that builds up that toxins are present and cause the body harm.

With regular cleaning of the tongue and good diet/exercise you can be sure the halitosis will be lessened and the anxiety it can cause will reduce.

CHAPTER 35

Zappicator and Syncrometer

These machines work by frequencies to kill off pathogens, chemicals and parasites from food, before they enter the body, and to get rid of them from the body when already ingested.

The syncrometer measures the level of parasites, which types are in which part of the body and the zappicator kills them off. As an opera singer would reach a frequency when the glass breaks, the same principle is applied to smashing parasites and chemicals.

Every living thing has its own frequency/vibration, these machines are programmed to kill them at these levels, causing no harm to the body, and the body's organs vibrate at a much higher level. Cleanses are then required to get rid of toxic debris from the kidneys, liver and skin.

These cleanses can be found commercially and naturally, thoroughly research any form of cleanse and consult your physician beforehand.

www.zappertek.com

Food and body zappicator

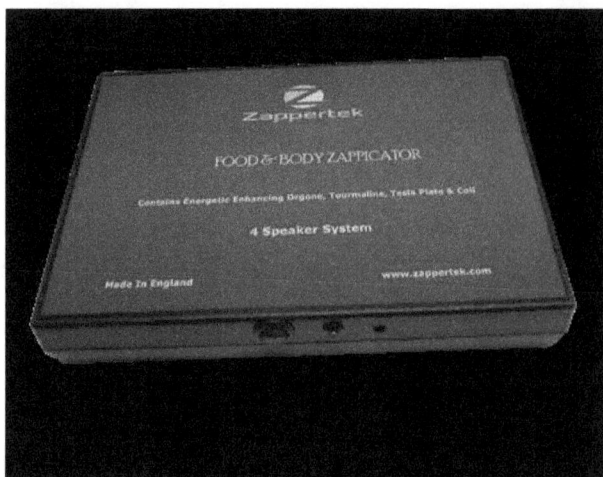

Tooth zappicator

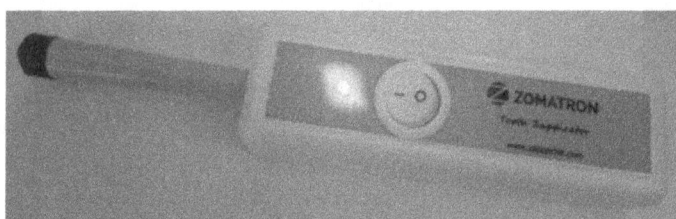

Can be used around the mouth, eyes, on the face, especially on spots and acne.

CHAPTER 36

The Powers of Juicing

The powers of juicing are amazing, reversing aging and illness, giving more energy, losing weight, curbing cravings, improving heart health, controlling diabetes, reducing anxiety, improving skin conditions, boosting mood, reducing pain and inflammation..

Juicing... fires up the immune system, oxygenates the body, energizes it, and neutralizing acidity.

Take all the nutrients from the live foods, and allow them to digest, taking pressure of the digestive tract and letting the body heal itself, see quickly how weight loss and increased energy happens, instead of impacted colon from bad foods(constipation)the body can concentrate on where it needs to be rather than fighting a losing gut battle. Recipes in part 3.

PART 3 - HEALTHY RECIPE OPTIONS

Introduction

So what can we eat??

After going through this book, you might be somewhat despondent with all the things you can't do...or shouldn't do, at least, if you want to lead a healthy life. There is good news! I have here for you a few nice recipes that you can use instead of buying packet stuff.

Making sure you wash all the ingredients in filtered water, magnetic is better, even if you do use tinned foods it will help to reduce , if not eliminate the chemicals and for the fresh foods, a must to wash it too, for pesticides and parasite removal, use a zappicator, mentioned in chapter 35 of part 2.

Eat a rainbow... eat all the colours of fresh foods you can find, each one is good for different things, yellow peppers, eggplant/aubergine, courgette/zucchini, red peppers, tomatoes, oranges, watermelon, cauliflower, just some examples.

Avoid using Teflon pans, Aluminium foil and be careful with the hygiene in the kitchen by cleaning cutting boards carefully, sterilizing equipment where possible to reduce bacterial infection.

Whereas vegetarian/vegan is better for detoxing your body and stresses the organs less when cleansing the digestive tract, meat takes three days to travel through the system, as do cheese and dairy products... aging the body through its extra pressure on liver/pancreas/gallbladder, bile ducts as they try to keep up with the whole cleansing process, when frying, use good oil, like coconut oil or olive oil.

Some of what you fancy does you good, but not to excess, for example fast food fries are double dipped in high fructose corn syrup and fried again to "enhance" crispiness and encourage you to eat more, the sugar/dopamine saga on the brain....reward system...it makes you want more!!

Some of the recipes do have sugar, but as alternatives to the packet junk we are exposed to nowadays, these are "wonder-foods" . Years ago Granny and Grandpa didn't get sick/ill, they lasted forever and told you stories of their younger days. They went to the store to buy a few things, came home and made stuff from scratch. Might have been high in calories in some cases but not loaded with preservatives and chemicals.

When I mention salt in these recipes I refer to Himalayan pink salt, kosher sea salt or similar, not table salt.

Healthy Snacks

Almonds, cranberries, walnuts, figs – all natural, unsalted, unsulphured, a handful every now and then helps stave off pangs of hunger and/or boredom... where high in nutrients be careful not to over eat as they are high in calories too.

Raw vegetables

Chopped up , prepared, ready to eat raw fruit and veg are always a good thing to have on hand to nibble from the fridge, kids love them too, cauliflower, broccoli, mini carrots, mushrooms, celery hearts, sliced apples, watermelon chunks, highly nutritious , full of vitamins and fibre...and great with a dip, make sure they are washed and cleaned before serving. Use a zappicator to reduce pathogen intake.

For information on the Zappicator check out: www.zappertek.com

Self-rising flour is not good, with its high GI index- which raises blood sugar levels, where possible use paleo, coconut or almond flour, there are many different flours, try them and see which is best for you.

Recipes

Carrot/ginger/sweet potato soup

Bag of carrots

Sweet potato- medium sized

2 inch piece of fresh ginger

Small onion

3 cloves of garlic

Head of broccoli

Black pepper to taste

Salt to taste

Turmeric 1 tsp.

Coriander 1 tsp.

4 cups of stock

Coconut oil 1 tbsp.

Coconut Milk 1x 8 oz tin

Method

Peel and dice all vegetables, add onion and garlic to spices and gently fry in oil until onion is tender. Add veg and stock. Bring to the boil, simmer for 30 minutes. Whizz with the blender. Add coconut milk and serve garnished with coriander sprigs of parsley.

Bean dip

2 x 8 oz. tins of butter beans (washed in filtered water) or 8 oz. of dry beans soaked in good water overnight and cooked for 2 hours before using.

Half a bulb of garlic, adjust to taste.

3 tablespoons of parsley

6 oz. of olive oil, adjust for constituency

Himalayan salt-1/2 teaspoon - according to taste

Method

Chop up garlic or whizz in a food processor.

Add beans, parsley, salt and olive oil and whizz again for a minute or so until all in a mixture.

Scrape out and chill in the fridge.

Spanish Omelette recipe

6 eggs- beaten

Potatoes- boiled and chopped into bite size pieces

Garlic – few cloves according to taste

Chopped onion

Salt to taste

Pepper to taste

Olive oil for frying

Method

Fry the onions and the garlic in a pan with olive oil until tender. Add the mix of potatoes, eggs, salt and pepper to the garlic and onion. Let cook gently, when browning, take a plate and flip it onto it by turning the pan upside down…whilst trying to keep all the bits together. Slide back into the pan to do the other side and cook all through the centre when browning again, turn out onto a plate, cut up and serve warm or cold from the fridge.

Biscuits/cookies/macaroons

8 oz flour – choices of almond/coconut /self-rising flour/paleo flour

Pinch of salt

5 oz. butter

4oz sugar

Vanilla -1 tablespoon- optional

Beaten egg to mix

Handful of raisins – optional

Method

Preheat oven to 350 f and grease baking tray

Add flour and salt, rub in butter, add sugar, mix to a dough with beaten egg and vanilla/raisins

Roll out onto a floured board and cut into cookie shapes or make balls of dough to form rock cakes...

Bake for 20 minutes in the centre of an oven or until pale gold.

Cornflake cakes

Cooking chocolate- dark, milk or white- 1 large bar

Chopped up figs or dates

8 oz. cornflakes

Large tablespoon of peanut butter

1 tablespoon of unsweetened coconut flakes

Colacao or drinking chocolate/cocoa powder- half a cup

Method

Mix all together in a large bowl, add to cake cases – leave in the freezer to chill. Ready to eat in half an hour

Scrambled eggs

4 eggs

Coconut oil

Himalayan Salt or sea salt (kosher)

Method

Beat eggs, add coconut oil and salt, add to pan and stir continuously for a few minutes.

Serve immediately

Fig Cake

3 cups chopped fresh figs

1 egg

2 cups of all-purpose flour/coconut/almond/paleo

1 cup of fat-free milk

1 cup of white sugar

1/4 cup of water

1 tablespoon of lemon juice

2 teaspoons of baking powder

1 teaspoon of vanilla extract

1/2 teaspoon of salt

1/4 cup of brown sugar

1/4 cup of butter

1/4 teaspoon of almond extract

Method

Take a bowl and mix the all-purpose flour, salt, and baking powder in it and keep it aside.

Preheat your oven to 175 C.

Take cake pans and spray vegetable oil on them.

Take another bowl and mix butter and sugar in it until the mixture turns fluffy.

Add eggs to it and beat well.

Add flour and milk to it.

Add vanilla essence, almond extract, and a cup of chopped figs to the bowl.

Pour this mixture into the pans and bake in the oven till you see the cake puffing.

Place a toothpick in the batter and bake till the toothpick comes out. This will take about 30 minutes. Take the cake out and let it cool.

To make a topping, take a pan and mix two cups of chopped figs, brown sugar, water, and lemon juice. Boil it until the paste thickens, which would take about 20 minutes. Spread the dough evenly onto the cake.

Scones/biscuits

12 oz. flour

½ level teaspoon salt

3 oz. butter/margarine

1 oz. sugar

¼ pint of milk

I level teaspoon of baking powder

Method

Add salt to the flour and rub in butter until it resembles breadcrumbs.

Add sugar

Add milk, mix to a soft but not sticky dough with a knife

Roll out and cut into 16-18 rounds with a 4-5cm cookie cutter

Bake in hot oven 450 f for 7-10 minutes or until golden brown

For cheese scones, omit the sugar and use ½ teaspoon of dry mustard, pinch of cayenne pepper and 4 oz. very finely grated cheese

Nut Roast

225g/8 oz Red lentils

2 cups/500ml Vegetable stock

1 Bay leaf

100g/4oz unsalted cashews

1 ½ tsp. olive oil

I large onion, finely chopped

1 large leek finely chopped

100g /4oz mushrooms chopped

1 or more cloves of garlic finely chopped or crushed

1 tablespoon of lemon juice

75 g /2 ½ oz. grated cheese

100g /4 oz. breadcrumbs

3 tablespoons chopped parsley

1 egg- beaten

Method

Mix together (bar the eggs and cheese) and cook in a pan. Tip the mix into a loaf pan and add cheese and beaten on top. Cover with foil and cook for 30 minutes remove foil and cook for another 30 minutes @ 350 F...

When cooked, pour over tomato sauce after slicing, allow to cool before slicing as it will crumble if sliced too hot.

Tomato sauce recipe

1 tablespoon tomato puree

½ teaspoon paprika

Tin of tinned tomatoes chopped

150 ml / 2/3 cup of stock

¼ tsp. mixed herbs

Method

Bring to the boil, add some extra cooked onion and then pour slowly over the loaf...

Cheese sauce

½ oz. Flour

½ oz. Butter/margarine/olive oil

Salt & Pepper

2 oz. Grated cheese

½ tsp. Mustard

½ pint Milk/water

Method

Melt butter/oil in a pan and mix with flour to a roux (doughy ball).

Add milk/water gradually stirring continuously with a whisk or spoon.

Add salt and pepper to taste, mustard and grated cheese...mix well and serve.

Salad and dressing

A variation of a healthy dressing, olive oil, mixed with Himalayan salt, Braggs ACV sprinkles over a mixture of spring mix, avocado, chopped cucumber, mushrooms, and spring onions.

Other ideas ...mashed cauliflower, quinoa, and couscous.

Carrot and apple juice

This not only tastes yummy but is very beneficial for boosting the immune system, aiding digestive system, colon health, protects eye health due to high vitamin A content, helps brain function, helps weight loss.

5 carrots, washed in filtered water

2 apples

Juice, chill and drink

You can help weight loss by substituting meals for juice, great for juice fasting too.

Kidney juice cleanse

2 apples

3½ watermelon pieces with rind, an inch a piece

Wash fruit well, juice and serve chilled, great for cleaning out the kidneys

Miracle skin

6 carrots

½ Green bell pepper

Wash well, juice and serve chilled...feeling those toxins leave your body, leaving you fresh clear skin.

Toxin flushes out

2 carrots

1 cucumber

½ cauliflower

½ beet

Cut stems off, unless organic, (chemicals are in the stems) wash well, juice and serve chilled.

Liver juice cleanse

½ beet with the greens

3 apples

Wash well, juice and serve chilled, great for cleaning out the liver after toxin build up, chemicals, parasites etc. Overload of the liver is easy to do, this will help shift things along.

There are many variations of juices that you can try that will help the body to cleanse itself and rejuvenate.

Garlic Mushrooms

Punnet of fresh whole mushrooms/sliced

2 cloves of garlic

Olive oil

Salt and pepper to taste

Herbs to taste

Method

Chop up mushrooms in bite sized pieces, fry in olive oil until tender and browning. Add salt, pepper and herbs. Serve immediately on a bed of rice or with toast, salad.

For a slight variation you can add a pinch of chili powder

Fried eggplant/aubergine

Thinly sliced eggplant/aubergine

Olive oil

Salt and pepper to taste

Method

Fry eggplant/aubergine in olive oil until browning, add salt and pepper, serve immediately as Hors d'oeuvre, or as a side veggie dish

Baked zucchini/courgette

4-6 large courgette/zucchini

Cream cheese to fill

Salt to taste

Olive oil

Method

Slice courgette/zucchini in half length-ways, cut flesh with a knife so cheese and oil soaks in...put cream cheese on top , drizzle olive oil over the whole thing and add salt. Bake in the centre of a moderate oven 375 F for 20-30 minutes, depending on size of veg or until cream cheese browns on top and the veg becomes tender and soft.

Honey nut Cookies

This recipe is even better as it has no sugar.

2 cups raw honey

4 cups almond flour

½ teaspoon nutmeg

½ teaspoon ginger

½ cup dried chopped dates

2 cups ground walnuts

½ cup of raisins

Method

Preheat the oven to 350 F.

Warm honey over low heat in a saucepan, allow to cool. Sift flour and spices. Add honey to the flour mix, stir well until blended. Stir in dates, walnuts and raisins...roll dough to ¼"thick, cut into squares.

Place squares on baking trays and cook for 10 minutes.

Banana bread

1 ¼ cups almond meal/flour

2 tsp. baking powder

¼ tsp. baking soda

½ cup fruit puree

¼ teaspoon cinnamon

½ teaspoon vanilla extract

2 large eggs

3 large ripe bananas, mashed

¼ cup flaxseed flour

½ cup chopped walnuts

½ cup unsweetened coconut flakes

Method

Preheat the oven to 350 F. In a large bowl, combine almond flour, baking powder, baking soda, puree, cinnamon and vanilla.

Add eggs, banana and flaxseed flour. Mix well

Add walnuts and coconut flakes, fold them into the mixture

Bake for 45 minutes

Ally's cookies

2 cups almond flour

½ cup coconut flour

½ teaspoon baking soda

1 tablespoon cinnamon

1 teaspoon dried ginger

½ teaspoon allspice

½ teaspoon nutmeg

¼ teaspoon cloves

1 cup raw honey

2 large eggs

1 tablespoon vanilla extract

¼ cup hazelnut flour

Method

Preheat oven 350 F/180 C

Mix almond flour, coconut flour, baking soda, cinnamon, ginger, allspice, nutmeg and cloves in a large bowl.

Add honey, eggs and vanilla to mix.

Add hazelnut flour and mix to form stiff dough.

Bake for 15 minutes

Add frosting - sandwich 2 cookies

4 tablespoons almond butter

2 tablespoons of raw honey

½ cup cacao nibs

½ tsp. Vanilla extract

½ tsp. cinnamon

Blend all ingredients well and whisk thoroughly. Ready to use!!!
Frosting can be used on any cake or cookies

Chocolate chip cookies

1 cup almond butter

2/3 cup shredded coconut

1 ½ tablespoons of coconut oil

1 cup cacao nibs

1/3 cup coconut flour

½ teaspoon cinnamon

1 egg

2 tablespoons cacao powder

½ cup raw honey

Method

Combine all the ingredients, mix well, make into ball shapes and
cook for 9 minutes at 350 F

Coconut cacao cookies

7 pitted dates

¾ cup almond flour

¼ cup coconut flour

½ cup shredded, unsweetened coconut

1 teaspoon coconut oil

2 tablespoons coconut milk

1 egg

1 cup cacao nibs

Method

Put dates and coconut into a food processor, pulse to a crumb like powder.

Pour mix into a large mixing bowl and add other ingredients, mix well with hands, make into balls or patties. Bake at 350F for 22 minutes

Toothpaste

All - natural toothpaste.

Cinnamon bark

Peppermint

Oregano

Stevia

Baking soda

Turmeric

Coconut oil

Neem oil

Method

Mix all together, keep in a non BPA container, glass is best...will harden when temperature is under 75 degrees Fahrenheit, use twice daily. Use peroxide and baking soda once a week too, and a tongue scraper daily, clean scraper in boiling water after each use.

Flu/cold remedy

Simple and effective.

Thyme oil, a few drops in a glass of water...will boost the immune system, oregano will also work.

Turmeric, ginger, garlic and honey in hot water will also remedy a cold and reduce sore throat and ache and pains.

Drink lots of pure water and juice to rid your body of toxic build up.

Super skin care routine

Wash your face with magnetized water every morning; this leaves the skin soft and supple, pat dry. Use apple cider vinegar toner diluted on a piece of cotton wool or flannel pat dry. Apply face cream, gently around the delicate eye area, patting rather than rubbing. Underneath makeup if you use it, use natural sunscreen if you go in the sun for UVA rays, also repels bugs.

Wash makeup off with magnetized water, use face scrub, (clears dead cells for renewal) wash off, pat dry and apply face cream.

Leaves skin like silk...

Use scrub on all of your body, especially elbows and feet to leave them supple and soft, pat dry and feel rejuvenated.

Keep skin hydrated, use a face sauna with distilled pure water, and use humidifiers throughout the house and bedroom, keeps airways clear too, especially in dry conditions, like heating in the winter will cause.

Drink lots of magnetised water to detox, reverse the sign of aging and wrinkles, has also been known to cure asthma a friend of mine had asthma for 30 years and by drinking magnetized water cures himself, makes the body highly charged, alkali, disease resistant, therefore disease cannot survive in the pure conditions.

****

Conclusion

Everyone has the choice to live in their world of toxins or to remove as many as possible from their lifestyle, breathing, eating and drinking. Begin your own journey of living in a toxin free household, no-one can help you if you won't help yourself, your animals and children. Remember... if your body gives you an illness or disease, think WHY? , detox a.s.a.p. If you get a cold, rest and don't eat, let your body detox and heal, allergies the same....it's all there for you to read...and inwardly digest.

Cures do not come in the form of a pill, a shot or some magical surgical procedure or treatment, allow your body to rest its organs and rid itself of toxins...it's a wonderful machine!!

READ LABELS - know what you are eating, drinking, putting on and in your skin and body. Remember... if you can't pronounce the name don't consume it.

Scurvy is simply a vitamin C deficiency and Osteoporosis a calcium deficiency we must remember. These diseases have been given names and treated to suppress the illness, not treat the cause.

The natural remedy for your condition must be personalised and customised based on finding the cause of your symptoms, illness and disease, then by reducing the intake of toxins from your daily routine as possible.

Not all diseases/illnesses are mentioned in this book, but on the whole you can be fairly certain that each and every one of them is because of pollutants and parasites. The body can become susceptible to depression and anxiety, creating a negative mind made worse by the negative company many people keep. Do not become the victim of a narcissist. They are very capable of turning an empathic person into their own breed of narcissists. See Brain Power by Miranda Carey- also available on Amazon.

The body is designed to rid itself of some toxins but not what we subject it to nowadays, air fresheners, cigarette smoke, vaping, pop, processed food, even shopping in a store, you risk toxic intake from bleached floors and air fresheners…etc. etc.

Reprogram your mind and body to live a different way, don't follow the "genetic" way and do what everyone else has done, living the same ways, eating the same foods, or you will end up with the "genetic" problem of your forefathers.

MY MISSION

The Ripple Effect messenger, if 1 person tells 10 people, they then, in turn, tell 10 people, bit by bit, it will make a huge difference.

Make people aware of what they are doing to their bodies, to stop the ongoing suffering of families and friends, to stop the unnecessary medical bills and drugs being taken. To make the world a healthier place. If only one person tells one person syndrome, that's great, to make everyone aware bit by bit, it can become possible,

POSITIVE IMPACT.

So try to forget what your forefathers told you, eat a huge whole hearty breakfast to get you through the day... WRONG! This leads to clogged up organs and leaves you feeling tired and even hungrier by mid-morning. Use autophagy (gentle fasting where your own body eats the bad cells) to optimize your health.

Eat if you feel unwell....WRONG! Your body doesn't need more toxins to get well, it needs NO toxins- Let organs/body get itself to pass all the yuck out, let the organs clean and do their job, have a break to repair the body... autophagy to rid your body of the bad stuff.

Sleep when your body tells you to sleep, it's the way it heals, and tells you to stop... slow down and sleep...do nothing. You detox whilst sleeping, your body's own mechanism for repairing.

Natural products, organic etc. cost more than your mass produced chemically based ones with preservatives and pesticides, but when you think about what you will save in health care and physical suffering, I think it's worth it.

Polluted, acidic bodies cause irreversible severe diseases - BE WARNED!

Accumulation of all ... .the straw that breaks the camel's back - you can live for a long time acidic but one extra toxin can break the whole body down.

Don't wait for the medical bills to come piling in.

Detox yourself, your mind and your environment NOW.

You can be well, it's up to you, make time.

You can afford it ...put back the convenience foods that pile up in the cupboard with sell by dates on, and buy fresh live foods...not tins and packets...filled with chemicals.

Glossary

Acidity- from being toxic can be from eating too much meat/ protein and not cleansing the body properly, from ingesting toxins that leave their waste in you, like parasites, and external chemicals from foods, cleaning products, airborne, personal care products, solvents, air fresheners.

Alkali- when your body is at the correct ph. level and is in harmony ...no disease can live in an alkaline body.

Anomaly - An anomaly is a pathogen that can affect your health, one that should not be in your body, such as bacteria, mold or fungi, parasites, stones etc.

Autophagy- Where your body's own cells eat the bad cells in your body by abstaining from eating for a length of time?

BPA / Bisphenol a - A chemical that is used in the making of plastic containers, make sure your drinking container is BPA free.

Carcinogenic - Cancer causing.

Detoxing - Eliminating toxins from the body.

Fasting - Abstaining from eating for a certain time. Different types of fast include juice fast, overnight fast, weekly/daily fast, 3-30 day fast.

Pathogen - An infectious being that causes disease such as bacteria, fungi, parasite, virus.

Vaping - Electronic cigarettes, vapourisers instead of smoking a cigarette, the process is known as to 'vape'

Disclaimer

Although everything in this book has been thoroughly researched, the information contained within must not be misconstrued as a cure or healing for any illness, a qualified physician must be consulted for any illness or disease and any treatment.

Further reading and references

Inspiration - A day at a time by Miranda Carey

Toxic 2 - The Carey formula by Miranda Carey

Toxic 3 - Brain Power by Miranda Carey

Hulda Regher Clark ...Cure for All Diseases/Cancers...

www.DrClarkStore.com

www.huldaclark.com

Bragg's Healthy Lifestyle and Miracles of Fasting

The Poisoned Planet by Timothy Oesch

The Fragrant Pharmacy by Valerie Ann Worwood

Fasting by Jentezen Franklin

The Art of Chi Kung by Wong Keiw Kit

Colon Health- The key to a vibrant life by Norman.W. Walker

The Hippocrates diet and health program by Ann Wigmore

Raw Energy by Leslie and Susannah Kenton

Dr Axe

Mercola.com

Livestrong.com

www.zappertek.com

Coming Soon... 'Toxic for Kids'

Preview of 'Toxic for Kids'

An easy to read guide for kids on toxic intake.

Ally asks...

What are we eating daily? What makes us ill? What's in a hot dog? What happens to you when you use the PC, tablet and TV? What causes anger and a bad attitude? What is autism and sleep apnea? What causes them? what's in our toilet roll? and shampoo? Mummy has cleaned the house again, what does that mean?

These are just some of the topics covered in 'Toxic for kids' to help both kids and their parents to understand why people get sick all the time without knowing how, and what they can do about it.

www.ingramcontent.com/pod-product-compliance
Lightning Source LLC
Chambersburg PA
CBHW050122280326
41933CB00010B/1205